WOMEN'S ISSUES

PRETERM BIRTH

PREVALENCE, RISK FACTORS AND MANAGEMENT

WOMEN'S ISSUES

Additional books and e-books in this series can be found on Nova's website under the Series tab.

WOMEN'S ISSUES

PRETERM BIRTH

PREVALENCE, RISK FACTORS AND MANAGEMENT

AGNITA MALIK
AND
ADAJA BAARDA
EDITORS

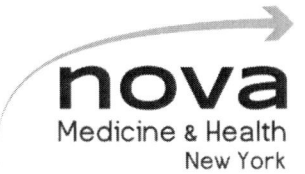

Copyright © 2020 by Nova Science Publishers, Inc.

All rights reserved. No part of this book may be reproduced, stored in a retrieval system or transmitted in any form or by any means: electronic, electrostatic, magnetic, tape, mechanical photocopying, recording or otherwise without the written permission of the Publisher.

We have partnered with Copyright Clearance Center to make it easy for you to obtain permissions to reuse content from this publication. Simply navigate to this publication's page on Nova's website and locate the "Get Permission" button below the title description. This button is linked directly to the title's permission page on copyright.com. Alternatively, you can visit copyright.com and search by title, ISBN, or ISSN.

For further questions about using the service on copyright.com, please contact:
Copyright Clearance Center
Phone: +1-(978) 750-8400   Fax: +1-(978) 750-4470   E-mail: info@copyright.com.

NOTICE TO THE READER

The Publisher has taken reasonable care in the preparation of this book, but makes no expressed or implied warranty of any kind and assumes no responsibility for any errors or omissions. No liability is assumed for incidental or consequential damages in connection with or arising out of information contained in this book. The Publisher shall not be liable for any special, consequential, or exemplary damages resulting, in whole or in part, from the readers' use of, or reliance upon, this material. Any parts of this book based on government reports are so indicated and copyright is claimed for those parts to the extent applicable to compilations of such works.

Independent verification should be sought for any data, advice or recommendations contained in this book. In addition, no responsibility is assumed by the Publisher for any injury and/or damage to persons or property arising from any methods, products, instructions, ideas or otherwise contained in this publication.

This publication is designed to provide accurate and authoritative information with regard to the subject matter covered herein. It is sold with the clear understanding that the Publisher is not engaged in rendering legal or any other professional services. If legal or any other expert assistance is required, the services of a competent person should be sought. FROM A DECLARATION OF PARTICIPANTS JOINTLY ADOPTED BY A COMMITTEE OF THE AMERICAN BAR ASSOCIATION AND A COMMITTEE OF PUBLISHERS.

Additional color graphics may be available in the e-book version of this book.

Library of Congress Cataloging-in-Publication Data

Names: Malik, Agnita, editor. | Baarda, Adaja, editor.
Title: Preterm birth : prevalence, risk factors and management / Agnita
   Malik, Adaja Baarda.
Description: New York : Nova Science Publishers, [2021] | Series: Women's
   issues | Includes bibliographical references and index. |
Identifiers: LCCN 2020030199 (print) | LCCN 2020030200 (ebook) | ISBN
   9781536182989 (paperback) | ISBN 9781536183504 (adobe pdf)
Subjects: LCSH: Premature labor. | Labor (Obstetrics)--Complications.
Classification: LCC RG649 .P7445 2021 (print) | LCC RG649 (ebook) | DDC
   618.3/97--dc23
LC record available at https://lccn.loc.gov/2020030199
LC ebook record available at https://lccn.loc.gov/2020030200

Published by Nova Science Publishers, Inc. † New York

CONTENTS

Preface		**vii**
Chapter 1	Epidemiological Factors for Preterm Birth: Maternal Factors *Panos Antsaklis, Maria Papamichail, Marianna Theodora and George Daskalakis*	**1**
Chapter 2	Epidemiological Factors for Preterm Birth: Paternal and Fetal Factors *Panos Antsaklis, Maria Papamichail, Marianna Theodora and George Daskalakis*	**45**
Chapter 3	The Link between DHA and Bone Turnover in the Preterm Neonate *Javier Diaz-Castro, Jorge Moreno-Fernandez and Julio J. Ochoa*	**57**
Chapter 4	Maternal Periodontal Disease and Adverse Pregnancy Outcomes: The Current Stand *Jananni Muthu and Sivaramakrishnan Muthanandam*	**79**
Index		**105**

PREFACE

Preterm birth is defined by WHO as birth before the 36 weeks and 6 days of gestation or before 259 days, counting from the first day of the last menstrual period. *Preterm Birth: Prevalence, Risk Factors and Management* presents an overview of the epidemiologic characteristics of women who deliver their neonates prematurely, in order to understand the depth of this major obstetrical problem.

Paternal risk factors, including paternal anthropometric and genetic characteristics and life-style habits, are addressed in conjunction with fetal characteristics which may be responsible for increasing the risk of preterm birth.

The authors discuss three important omega-3 fatty acids for the prevention of osteopenia of the preterm newborn: alpha-linolenic acid, eicosapentaenoic acid, and docosahexaenoic acid.

The concluding study explores the mechanisms that link periodontitis with adverse pregnancy outcomes and presents a comprehensive critical review of the current scientific stand regarding this relationship.

Chapter 1 - Preterm birth is defined by WHO as birth before the 36 weeks and 6 days of gestation or before 259 days, counting from the first day of the last menstrual period. Preterm birth can be sub-grouped based on gestational age as: extremely preterm birth (less than 28 weeks), very preterm (31-28 weeks), moderate to late preterm birth (32-37 weeks) or based on the cause of preterm birth as: spontaneous preterm birth with intact membranes, premature rupture of the membranes leading to preterm birth and indicated preterm birth due to maternal or fetal medical conditions. The latest rates of preterm birth published show that in 2014 preterm birth rate was 8.7% in Europe, while in Africa was 13.4%, estimating that 15 million babies were born preterm globally for that year. Preterm births are responsible for 65-75% of neonatal deaths and up to 75% of neonatal morbidity and contribute to long-term neurocognitive deficits, pulmonary dysfunction and ophthalmologic disorders. Despite the enormous progress made in neonatal medicine, leading to major increase of survival of the very-preterm babies, preterm birth complications are responsible for 1 million deaths among children younger than 5 five years. The aim of this chapter is to present an overview of the epidemiologic characteristics of women who deliver their neonates prematurely, in order to get to the depth of this major obstetrical problem and help to the better understanding of preterm labour, in order to get closer to the solution. Risk factors include maternal demographic characteristics (e.g., age, race-ethnicity, educational level, income and marital status), maternal behaviour such as smoking or alcohol consumption, obstetric history and complications.

Chapter 2 - Preterm birth is a global subject of interest, as WHO estimated that in 2014 more than 15 million neonates were born prematurely. Despite the enormous progress in neonatology, preterm birth remains a major obstetrical problem, being responsible for 65 - 75% of neonatal deaths and 75% of neonatal morbidity. Preterm birth has been characterized as an obstetrical syndrome, with multifactorial etiology and multiple pathophysiological mechanisms, in which the immune system and its responses playing a major role. In order to decrease the incidence of preterm birth and therefore to limit its consequences, it is important to try and understand this syndrome from an epidemiologic point of view, to detect the risk factors and when possible to avoid them. In the past years, maternal risk factors for preterm delivery were the most studied ones. However, some important risk factors concerning either the fetal or the paternal side, have been proved to be equally important. In this chapter, the authors will review the paternal risk factors including paternal anthropometric and genetic characteristics and life-style habits. In addition, fetal characteristics which may be responsible for increasing the risk of preterm birth will be discussed, including fetal sex, congenital anomalies and complications (i.e., severe I.U.G.R, fetal distress).

Chapter 3 - According to the World Health Organization, 10% of the world's births occur before the 37th week of gestation. A significant increase in the survival rate of preterm infants has been reported in recent decades. In parallel, this has increased emerging conditions, such as osteopenia of prematurity, which can occur in up to 30% of infants born before the 28th week of gestation. The prevalence depends on gestational age, weight and type of diet. It occurs in 55% of premature babies weighing less than 1,000 g and in 23% of infants weighing less than 1,500 g at birth. Osteopenia of the newborn is characterized by the reduction of bone mineral content, and is caused both by severe nutritional deficiencies and by biomechanical factors. It occurs between the tenth and sixteenth weeks of life, but may not be detected until there is severe demineralization (between 20 and 40% loss of bone mineral). Despite being a common disease, there are important controversies in the literature regarding the methods of detection of infants at risk, as well as their interpretation. The prevention of osteopenia of the preterm newborn and its timely treatment should be the primary objective of health. In this sense, ω-3 polyunsaturated fatty acids (ω-3 PUFA) are a group of fatty acids (FA) that are essential components of the human diet because they cannot be synthesized. Three important omega-3 fatty acids are alpha-linolenic acid (ALA), eicosapentaenoic acid (EPA), and docosahexaenoic acid (DHA). Sources of EPA and DHA are fatty fish such as salmon, fish oil supplements, or the conversion of ingested alpha-linolenic acid to DHA or EPA, though evidence reports that the conversion rate is low, especially in the neonate. ω-3 PUFA play an important role in bone metabolism and may represent a useful non-pharmacological way of ameliorating bone loss and risk of osteoporosis. ω-3 is precursor for several potent regulatory eicosanoids involved in bone metabolism including PG and leukotrienes. Thereby, ω-3 PUFA can inhibit the production of these inflammatory cytokines such as IL-1, IL-6 and TNF-α, which provide an important stimulus for osteoclastic bone resorption, and suppression of the production of these cytokines by n-3 PUFA may inhibit bone resorption and prevent bone loss.

Chapter 4 - Periodontitis is a multifactorial chronic inflammatory disease of the supporting structures of the tooth, which when untreated can result in loss of function of the teeth and eventually tooth loss. The primary etiology for periodontal disease is the bacterial pathogens that evoke a host inflammatory response. The host bacterial interaction is not only localized to the oral cavity but also evokes systemic response elsewhere in the body. In the few past decades chronic periodontal disease has been linked to various systemic diseases like cardiovascular diseases, diabetes mellitus, respiratory illnesses, renal diseases and adverse pregnancy outcomes, leading to the emergence of a new branch of periodontology known as periodontal medicine. Adverse pregnancy outcomes represent an important health issue which affects not only the infant but also the mother. There is evidence that adverse pregnancy outcomes are correlated with intra-uterine infections and increased local and systemic inflammatory markers. Periodontitis being a chronic inflammatory disease might contribute to this systemic inflammation. The most common adverse pregnancy outcomes that have been associated with chronic periodontal disease are premature rupture of membranes and preterm birth, low birth weight, and preeclampsia. Research in the past few years have established periodontal disease as a risk factor for adverse pregnancy outcomes and studies have also proved that treatment of periodontal disease reduced the risk for adverse pregnancy outcomes. This paper aims in exploring the mechanisms that link periodontitis with adverse pregnancy outcomes and also presents a comprehensive critical review of the current scientific stand regarding this relationship.

In: Preterm Birth
Editors: A. Malik and A. Baarda
ISBN: 978-1-53618-298-9
© 2020 Nova Science Publishers, Inc.

Chapter 1

EPIDEMIOLOGICAL FACTORS FOR PRETERM BIRTH: MATERNAL FACTORS

Panos Antsaklis, MD, PhD, Maria Papamichail*, MD, Marianna Theodora, MD, PhD and George Daskalakis, MD, PhD

1st Department of Obstetrics and Gynecology,
Department of Fetal Maternal Medicine,
Alexandra Maternity Hospital, University of Athens,
Athens, Greece

ABSTRACT

Preterm birth is defined by WHO as birth before the 36 weeks and 6 days of gestation or before 259 days, counting from the first day of the last menstrual period. Preterm birth can be sub-grouped based on gestational age as: extremely preterm birth (less than 28 weeks), very preterm (31-28 weeks), moderate to late preterm birth (32-37 weeks) or based on the cause of preterm birth as: spontaneous preterm birth with intact membranes, premature rupture of the membranes leading to

---

* Corresponding Author's E-mail: mapapam@hotmail.com.

preterm birth and indicated preterm birth due to maternal or fetal medical conditions. The latest rates of preterm birth published show that in 2014 preterm birth rate was 8.7% in Europe, while in Africa was 13.4%, estimating that 15 million babies were born preterm globally for that year. Preterm births are responsible for 65-75% of neonatal deaths and up to 75% of neonatal morbidity and contribute to long-term neurocognitive deficits, pulmonary dysfunction and ophthalmologic disorders. Despite the enormous progress made in neonatal medicine, leading to major increase of survival of the very-preterm babies, preterm birth complications are responsible for 1 million deaths among children younger than 5 five years. The aim of this chapter is to present an overview of the epidemiologic characteristics of women who deliver their neonates prematurely, in order to get to the depth of this major obstetrical problem and help to the better understanding of preterm labour, in order to get closer to the solution. Risk factors include maternal demographic characteristics (e.g., age, race-ethnicity, educational level, income and marital status), maternal behaviour such as smoking or alcohol consumption, obstetric history and complications.

Keywords: epidemiology of preterm birth, maternal risk factors

1. INTRODUCTION

Preterm birth is defined by WHO as live birth before 36^{+6} weeks of gestation or as a pregnancy length shorter than 259 days, counting from the first day of the last menstrual period [1]. The survival rate of preterm babies has been significantly increased, due to the evolution of obstetrics and neonatology. Therefore, the very good survival rate of neonates born after 34 weeks has led some specialists to suggest that preterm birth definition should be redefined as the birth before the 34th week of gestation [2].

The definition of preterm birth is difficult as not only the gestational age up to which a neonate is considered preterm has been questioned, but mainly the definition of the lower limit, the limit of the so called viability, is an area of great discussion among neonatologists and obstetricians. Different laws, religious and cultural customs and of course potential of neonatal units have led to different definitions of the limit of viability in different countries. Lumley et al. [3] noticed in their survey, that if all births between 20-23 weeks of gestation are considered as spontaneous abortion and they are not counted as preterm births, then the preterm birth rate will be decreased by 4%. Studies that took place in the beginning of the millenium, suggested that the lower limit of preterm birth should be between 23-24th gestational week, which corresponds to a fetal weight of 500 kilograms [4-5].At this point is necessary to mention the importance of correct dating of the pregnancy, as gestational age should be confirmed ideally in the first trimester.

Chawanpaiboon et al. [1] searched data from all around the world concerning preterm birth rates, for a 25 year period, from 1990 to 2014. They found that preterm birth rate has been increased from 9.8% in 2000 to 10.6% in 2014. In numbers, 14.84 million babies were born prematurely during 2014, while 81.1% of these, were born in sub-Saharan Africa and Asia. The highest preterm birth rate was identified in North Africa (13.4%) and the lowest in Europe (8.7%), with India having the leading part in global preterm birth rates, as they are responsible for 23.4% of all preterm births occurring around the world.

Preterm birth is considered as the major obstetrical problem and this is due to the fact that preterm birth is responsible for 65-75% of neonatal deaths and 75% of neonatal morbidity [6,7], affecting not only the new borns and their families, but also their social environment. Preterm birth is the leading cause for neonatal death in the first month of a neonate's life and the second cause of mortality among children under-5-years of age [8]. More than one million babies died as a direct result of their prematurity in 2010 [9], while at the same time, complications of prematurity such as infections are responsible for more than one million of deaths of premature newborns regardless of the cause that led to preterm birth [10]. Interestingly, even for neonates that have been born at the 32-34th week of gestation and are considered to have optimal survival rate, increased morbidity is present until their first year of life, mainly due to respiratory complications, infections and the neonatal sudden death syndrome [11]. Unfortunately, preterm birth accompanies for a lifetime a significant percentage of the babies that have been born prematurely, as disability and complications, such as neurodevelopmental impairments, learning difficulties, respiratory and gastrointestinal complications affects their late-teen and adult life [7].

2. MATERNAL RISK FACTORS

Preterm birth is a major obstetrical problem with severe consequences to the newborn itself, its parents, their social cycle and finally the healthcare and government expenditure. A very important issue is to identify women at risk for preterm birth, in order to offer her the optimal prenatal care and health advice and under these circumstances decrease her possibility of preterm birth. This is why it is important for obstetricians to study and identify the potential risk factors for preterm birth as soon as possible, even before conception and aim to modify them.

2.1. Recurrent Preterm Birth

Obstetric history and more specifically preterm birth is the most powerful factor predisposing to preterm birth. Philips et al. [13] in their meta-analysis found that the absolute risk for recurrent preterm birth for women with at least one previous preterm birth is 30%. This percentage differs according to the mechanism of preterm birth: for premature rupture of the membranes (PROM) the recurrence risk is 7%, while for premature labor the risk is 23%. In a recent meta-analysis [14], the overall risk of recurrence in women with previous preterm was smaller (20.2%). Moreover, the gestational age when the previous preterm birth had occurred, is also related to the possibility of recurrence, with women delivering prior to 32 weeks of gestation to having a greatest risk, compared to those who delivered after 32 weeks. Additionally, the risk of recurrence is increasing as the gestational week of previous delivery decreases. More specifically, preterm birth prior to 32 weeks had 23.3 OR to give childbirth before 32 gestational weeks, 9.2 OR to deliver between

32-36 weeks and 1.9 OR to deliver at early term (37-38 weeks), when compared to women delivering at 39 weeks or further [18]. This pattern was also noticed in women who had their previous delivery at early term. Their possibility to deliver prior to 32 weeks was 2 times higher, 3 times higher to deliver between the 32nd and the 36th gestational week and 2.2 times higher to delivery between the 37 and 38 week compared to women who delivered at term (39 weeks or further). Additionally, it was suggested that a spontaneous previous preterm birth could also be related to an increased possibility of medically indicated preterm birth or vice versa [17]. The fact that the obstetrical history is one of the most sensitive factors that can increase the possibility of preterm birth, indicates that genetics might have a significant role on the mechanisms leading to premature delivery. Interestingly sisters and daughters of women who had recurrent preterm births, presented also increased possibilities for preterm birth [19].

However, it has been argued that anxiety could be the factor that increases the risk of preterm birth rather than genetic background, as many women with a previous preterm birth are more anxious in the current pregnancy, worrying about the outcome. As it will be discussed further below, anxiety is another factor increasing the possibilities for preterm birth [15-16].

2.2. Uterine Anomalies

Congenital anomalies of the uterusand mainly major anomalies, namely uterine duplication, didelphys, bicornuate, unicornuate uterus or mullerian abnormalities have been considered responsible for preterm birth [20-22]. Nevertheless, minor abnormalities such as arcuate uterus, septate or t-shape uterus where a midline septum is present provoking minimal fundal cavity indentation, can also increase the risk of preterm birth. Therefore, concerning uterine anomalies, women must be sub-grouped according to the type of the anomaly [21]. Fox et al. in their survey found that 50% of patients with unicornuate uterus delivered prematurely. The percentage for bicornuate, didelphys, not repaired septate, repaired septate t-shaped and arcuate uterus were 39%, 33%, 25%, 16%, 20% and 7% respectively.

Uterine fibroids are very common among women of reproductive age and they can be present up to 3-12% of pregnant women [23]. Uterine fibroids and more specifically large or intramular fibroids are responsible for increased risk for preterm birth. Klatsky et al. [24] in their meta-analysis reported that 16% of women with fibroids would deliver prematurely, showing similar results with recent studies, which showed that about 10% of pregnant women with uterine fibroids will give birth prematurely [25-27]. This means that women with fibroids have 2 times higher risk of preterm birth compared to general population. The size of the fibroids is related to the time of delivery: women with fibroids 5 cm or less, delivered at median gestational age of 38.4 weeks while women with fibroids larger than 5 cm delivered significantly earlier (median gestational age 36.5 weeks) [28]. When the location of the fibroids is concerned, there is no difference between pregnancy outcome between fibroids located in the posterior or the anterior uterine wall [29]. Additionally, the presence of multiple fibroids increases significantly the risk for preterm birth compared to single fibroids [30]. Aprecise explanation of the mechanism that a fibroid can cause preterm birth is difficult to be set. One theory suggests that degenerating fibroids irritate the myometrium resulting to premature uterine contractions and cervical change or ripening. Moreover, fibroid uterus shows a decreased oxytocinase activity, leading to higher concentrations of oxytocin, predisposing again to premature contractions [31].

2.3. Interpregnancy Interval

Interpregnancy interval (IPI) is defined as the period between the delivery of a previous pregnancy and conception of the next pregnancy. Both small and long interpregnancy intervals are associated with higher risk for preterm birth following a U-shaped analogy.

Many trials run in the past decade, showed that women with interpregnancy intervals less than 6 months, had 30-90% higher risk for preterm birth [32-33]. More recent trials, confirmed these data, as in 2018 Hegelundet al. [36] found that women with IPI of 0 to 5 months have 22.4 more preterm births per 1000 live births, compared to women with IPI of 18-23 months. Additionally, Conde-Agudelo [40] et al., in their meta-analysis demonstrated that women with IPI shorter than 6 months have 40% higher risk for preterm birth compared to women with IPI of 18 months or longer. However, it has been noticed that women with short interpregnancy intervals are usually women with complications in their last pregnancy and also have socio-demographics characteristics that increase their risk of preterm birth and other pregnancy complications [33]. The theory explaining the higher possibility for adverse perinatal outcomes in short interpregnancy intervals is the "maternal nutritional depletion syndrome," suggesting that the mother does not have the time to recover from childbirth and breastfeeding and her nutrient stores are insufficient to manage another pregnancy [34].

In contrast, a survey published in 2019, suggests that interpregnancy intervals longer than 120 months increase the risk for premature rupture of the membranes [35]. This fact that is coming to agreement with Hegelund et al. [36] findings, demonstrating that women with interpregnancy intervals longer than 60 months have 13.1 times higher risk of preterm births per 1000 live births, compared to women with interpregnancy intervals of 18-23 months. The explanation for this finding is that women might lose the advantage of physiological adaption to pregnancy and delivery [36].

The ideal interpregnancy interval with the lowest risk of preterm birth, has been calculated between 18-36 months. For this period (18-36 months) the longer the interpregnancy interval, the lower the risk for preterm birth, so that the ideal period would be after 18 months but closer to 36 months [37]. WHO after considering these facts, recommends that interpregnancy interval should be 2 years or longer [38].

2.4. Cervical Length

It is commonly accepted by the obstetrician community that cervical length (CL) is one of the strongest factors responsible for spontaneous preterm birth [43]. The measurement of the cervical length by transvaginal ultrasound became a routine in the second trimester. A cervix shorter than 25mm is consider as "short" as it corresponds to the 10th percentile for the current gestational age [41]. Additionally, for every increase of cervical length beyond 25mm, the possibility for preterm birth is decreased by 6% (OD: 0.91) [42].Owen et al. [41] came in opposite results as they found that the absolute length of the cervix above 25mm has limited impact on the risk for preterm birth and it is remain stable at 16% for every measurement above 25 mm. Moreover, the earlier in pregnancy a short cervix is identified, the higher the risk for preterm birth; the risk for preterm birth is declined by 5% for every week of detection of CL <25mm after the 18th week of gestation. Among women in high risk for preterm birth due to their obstetric history, without symptoms of premature labor and with cervical length shorter than 25mm, the incidence for delivering prematurely is 2.5 times higher than asymptomatic, high-risk women with CL > 25mm [41].

The last decade, many articles occupied with the impacts of procedures for the treatment of cervical intraepithelial neoplasia (CIN), as women who must undergo to these procedures, have the same age with women having their first child [49]. Since the 1980s, surveys claimed that surgical cervical conization rises the possibility for preterm birth [44-46], with more recent trials with larger patient numbers confirming these results [47-48]. Furthermore, the risk for preterm birth is increasing for every increase on cone depth excision [49]. More specifically, compared to women with no cervical intervention, women with cone depth excision of 10-12mm had 1.5 times higher risk for preterm birth, 2.77 and 4.91 times higher risk for cone depth excision of 15-17mm and over 20mm respectively [49]. The multiple treatments also rise the risk for preterm birth for about 4 times. Additionally, the innovating procedures which have been introduced for CIN treatment limit the effect of these procedures on the risk for preterm birth, but not that sharply. Namely, for cold knife conization the risk is 2.7 times higher [50], for abliative treatment the risk is 1.35 times higher, for laser conization 2 times higher and for loop excision 1.58 times higher.

2.5. Previous Miscarriage and Pregnancy Termination

Medical interventions following a miscarriage or pregnancy termination have the potential to increase the risk for preterm birth. Women with one or two spontaneous miscarriages, or pregnancy terminations are generally considered higher risk for preterm birth, however this has been disputed when these women receive the proper antenatal care [51]. Virk et al. [52] run a trial including almost 12000 pregnant women and they concluded that one previous miscarriage or pregnancy termination irrespectively of the medical technique used, does not increase the risk for preterm birth. McCarthy et al. [51] confirmed the previous data, as in their study they calculated miscarriages and pregnancy terminations as 'pregnancy losses' and the risk for preterm birth was not increased compared to women with no pregnancy losses. In contrast, women with one previous termination of pregnancy had slightly increased risk for preterm birth (OD: 1.48) [51]. Oliver-Williams et al. [53] concluded that the association between a previous miscarriage was stronger for the extreme preterm birth (24-28 weeks of gestation). McCarthy et al. [51] noticed that for women with two previous miscarriages, the risk for delivering prematurely was 2 to 3 times higher (PPROM OD: 3.31, sPTB OD: 3.14), compared to women with no pregnancy loses [51, 53]. Moreover, Oliver-Williams et al. showed an 18% increase in the odds of spontaneous preterm birth for each previous pregnancy termination, while the risk for induced preterm labor remained the same and similar to women who had no history of pregnancy loses.

Concerning the medical technique used to treat a miscarriage, cervical dilatation and curettage was associated with a 60% increased risk for preterm birth for women with one pregnancy loss, while for women having two or three pregnancy losses managed by cervical dilatation and curettage, the risk for preterm birth was more than two times higher (OD:2.32) [51].

2.6. Maternal Age

According to many surveys, extreme maternal age, either very young (15-18 years) or advanced maternal age (≥ 40 years) is associated with a higher risk of preterm birth [5], and it follows a U-shaped association. The 21st century is characterized by the social equality of women and the increase of the artificial reproductive technologies, resulting to women achieving pregnancies at advanced age. Recent data, estimated that the percentage of women who gave birth after 45 years of age, was 0.05-0.2% [54]. It is reasonable that advanced maternal age bares risks, but on the other hand pregnancy at that stage is associated with wealthier income and higher socio-economic status [55]. It is well known that advancing maternal age increases the risk of pregnancy complications such as gestational diabetes, hypertension and pre-eclampisa in addition to pre-existing disorders. For women older than 45 years, the risk for delivering prematurely before the 37 weeks is 1.5 to 3.0 times greater and 2.0-3.0 times greater for preterm birth before the 32 weeks. Eliyahu et al. [5] run a trial including 17000 pregnant women and they concluded that women aged over 45 years presented the highest risk for preterm birth, with their risk increasing up to 20%. For women between 16 and 20 years the risk was 12.5%, 8% for women aged 21-40 years and 14.2% for women in the 41-45 age group. Lowler et al. [55] showed that the lowest rates of preterm birth are found in women aged 24-30 years and the highest in women older than 35 years, but with smaller percentages (5% for the 20-29 age group and 7% for the >35 years age group). Furthermore, Goisis et al. [57] in their cohort found that women older than 40 years had almost three times greater rates for delivering prematurely, when compared to women in the 24-30 age group. Additionally, women older than 40 years had twice greater rates for iatrogenic preterm birth, due to medical conditions. Fuchs et al. [56] concluded that the lowest preterm birth rates were found in the group of women aged between 30 - 34 years. Interestingly, Khahil et al. [58] found no proofs that advanced maternal age is related to higher risk for preterm birth.

Concerning the other extreme age group, teen pregnancy carries also greater risk for preterm birth, mainly due to gynecological immaturity and nutritional insufficiency [55].Additionally, the socio-economic status of teen mothers tends to be less favorable than pregnancy in older ages. In contrast to the pregnant women of advanced maternal age who deliver prematurely due to iatrogenic reasons and have higher rates of induction of labor, teen mothers tend to have higher rates for spontaneous preterm birth [56]. Avezedo et al. [59-62] in their review showed that adolescent pregnancy (maternal age <19 years) had 2 times higher risk (OD: 1.77-2.07) for preterm birth compared to mothers aged from 20 to 29 years old.

2.7. Artificial Reproductive Technologies (ART)

As it is mentioned above, artificial reproductive technologies have been rapidly increasing the past two decades, resulting to higher prevalence of multiple pregnancies. ART is responsible for 21% of all twin and triplet pregnancies and for the 66% of the increase in preterm birth rates globally. Kashnir et al. [63] counted the risk for preterm birth among infants born via ART and found that for all ART procedures, the rates of preterm birth were 16.5% for singletons, 63.9% for twins and 100% for triplets. Interestingly, when comparing multiple gestations achieved after spontaneous conception and after ART, multiple pregnancy after ART showed greater risk for preterm birth. Additionally, ART increases the risk for pregnancy complications and more specifically preterm birth before the 33rd gestational week. Helmershort et al. [64] concluded that the risk for premature birth before the 32nd week was 3.27, while the same risk was 2.07 for preterm birth before the 37th gestational week.

Women with subfertility problems have greater risk of obstetric complications including preterm birth, even when no treatment is given or when the outcome of the artificial reproductive technologies is a singleton pregnancy [65]. This can be explained by pre-existing disorders which in general are more frequent in this group of women, including uterine abnormalities or pelvic infection and consequences of the infertility management, including the diagnostic or therapeutic - operative procedures. Perri et al. [66] concluded that women undergoing intracytoplasmic sperm injection (ICSI) due to subfertility of their partner, the risk for preterm birth was equal to women without subfertility problems. Henriksen et al. [67] in their research concluded that the risk of preterm birth is increasing progressively with the increase of waiting time to pregnancy, regardless of the infertility treatment [68]. Weng et al. [69] showed that when women undergo low-tech procedures (namely intrauterine insemination and ovulation induction) did not present greater risk for preterm birth, when compared to women who had spontaneous conception. In contrast, women who achieved pregnancy through high-tech techniques such as in vitro fertilisation (IVF), intracytoplasmic sperm injection (ICSI) or gamete intrafallopian transfer (GIFT), the risk for delivering prematurely before 32 weeks of gestation, was significantly higher comparing to the control group.

2.8. Multiple Gestations

Although multiple gestations represent 1-3% of all pregnancies, they are responsible for 12-33.7% of preterm births globally [70-71]. In an effort to explain the reasons why multiple pregnancies have higher risk for preterm birth, uterine overdistension, uterine ischemia, hormonal disorders and abnormal allograft reaction are some of the most popular theories that have been discussed [77]. It is estimated that 50% of twin pregnancies result in premature delivery, 10% of preterm twin infants are born before the 28th gestational week and another 10% of them are born between the 28th and the 31st gestational week [17]. Martin et al. [72] concluded that twin pregnancies had 12 times greater risk for preterm birth compared to singleton pregnancies. The rates for preterm birth for twin pregnancies for the 37th, the 34th and the 32nd week are 41%, 13% and 7%, respectively

[73].The median gestational age of delivery for twin pregnancies is the 36th week. A factor that plays significant role for the risk of preterm birth is chorionicity: monochorionic twins have greater risk for being born prematurely, compared to dichorionic twins [74]. Breathnachet al. [75] claimed that 34% of monochorionic twins are born before the 34th week of gestation, while the 29% of dichorionic twins are born before the 36thgestational week. Concerning triplet pregnancies, more than 90% of triplet infants are born prematurely [76], while the median gestational age for delivery for triplet pregnancies is the 33rd gestational week.

2.9. Number of Gestations

Preterm birth occurs more frequently in nulliparous women and the risk tends to be reduced with every new pregnancy [78]. Despite the fact that many trials claimed that the greater the number of gestations, the greater the risk for preterm birth, there were doubts about their validation and it was proved that the risk for preterm birth is reduced for every new pregnancy and this analogy is valid until the fourth pregnancy [79]. There are only a few trials identifying the risk for preterm birth after the fourth pregnancy. Eliyahu et al. [5] in their study included 17497 births, dividing women in two groups: women with 8 pregnancies or more and women with less than 8 pregnancies. The preterm birth rate in the first group was greater compared to the second group: 13.8 and 8.5% respectively. Nevertheless, it appears that multiparous women tend to have advanced age and their socio-economic status tends to be less favorable, setting doubts about the correlation with multiparity as an independent risk factor for preterm birth [80].

2.10. Socio-Economic Status

It has been proved that among populations with low socio-economic status, the risk for preterm birth is greater. Byrne and Morrison claimed that low-socio-economic status in combination with previous preterm birth are the two strongest risk factors for preterm birth [81]. Socioeconomic factors are related to the life style, occupation, income, educational level and all together constitute strong risk factors for preterm birth [82]. Although the mechanisms for this relation have not been verified yet, the young age of these women, maternal health behaviors resulting to insufficient antenatal care, the higher prevalence of tobacco, alcohol and drugs usage during pregnancy, the insufficient nutritional intake, the increased frequency of urinary truck infections and sexually transmitted diseases and the higher prevalence of psychological disorders presenting in women in lower socioeconomic levels, are some points that might explain why preterm birth presents higher rates in this population. Hegelund et al. [81] calculated that women with low educational attainment experienced 1.3 more preterm births per 1000 live births compared to women with higher educational level. Another important factor related to the socioeconomic position is income, which is often determined by educational level [83-84]. Women of poorer economical background and of black ethnicity are more likely to deliver prematurely than wealthier women with the same race (12.2% *vs* 7.4% respectively).

2.11. Race – Ethnicity

Many surveys mainly from U.S.A., suggest that the incidence of preterm birth is higher among Black and Hispanic women. In addition, studies from other developed countries concluded that women coming from minority racial groups, had greater risk for preterm birth compared to local women. Preterm birth rate for African-American women was 18,4%, while the same rate for non-Hispanic White women was 11.7% [85]. Data show that infants of black women have a 50% greater possibility to be born prematurely, compared to non-black infants [82], meaning that black women have two-fold increased risk for delivering prematurely [85-86]. Additionally, black infants that are born prematurely, have shorter gestational duration compared to premature white infants. Non-Hispanic

Black women have a 4 times higher risk for recurrent preterm birth and 6.4 times higher risk for premature rupture of membranes. Concerning Asian races, different studies show conflicting results: some of them concluded that Asian women do not carry a greater risk for preterm birth compared to non-Hispanic White women, while other studies show that they have a greater risk for preterm delivery [93]. When further analysis divided Asian races in 'East" and 'South' Asian, among East Asian population, the risk for preterm birth was equal to Caucasian population, while among South Asian population, the risk for both iatrogenic and spontaneous preterm birth was found to be greater compared to Caucasian women. Finally, Afro-Caribbean women and women from mixed racial origin were more likely to deliver prematurely due to iatrogenic interventions, mainly induction to labor.

The significance of the effect of racial disparities on preterm birth, is that this effect persist even after accounting for known preterm birth risk factors such as smoking, maternal education level, and socio-economic status. Racial and ethnic differences in allele frequencies may have a key-role to these disparities [87]. Many studies confirm that there is a clear familiar relationship to preterm birth; women with a first degree relative who delivered prematurely, present higher risk for preterm birth. Inflammation genes might also have an association with preterm birth; in a large study, researchers identified seven genes that increase the risk for preterm birth among African-American women involving inflammation, extracellular remodeling and cell signaling. The gene with the strongest correlation with preterm birth is the protein kinase C-alpha (PRKCA) gene [88]. Additionally, epigenetics with the gene activity and expression modification, could also explain the hereditability of preterm birth. Three trials studied the CpG methylation of the genome and concluded that there were differences between the cord blood of premature and term infants, suggesting that the lower the genome methylation, the lower the gestational duration [89-91]. Finally, although placental telomere length of African-American women was significant lower than White Women, it a clear correlation to perinatal outcomes could not be proven [92].

2.12. Environmental Exposure

Environmental exposure factors such as air pollution and toxins, contaminated water, pesticides, traffic density and household hygiene are shown to have association with preterm birth, probably through mechanisms such as oxidative stress and inflammation [94-98]. Williams and Collins [99] in their trial suggested that residential segregation leads to disparities in health through "pathogenic residential conditions." Black and poorer families are more likely to live in abandoned buildings and more commercial and industrial facilities, to have unhealthy housing quality with high noise levels, exposure to allergens (e.g., dust mites), pollutants (e.g., particulates) and lead. Additionally, poorer households are often overcrowded, as a lot of people have to survive in tiny spaces. Concerning lead exposure, its correlation with preterm birth has been established since 1994, when Andrews et al. [100] in their study found that women who had delivered prematurely had higher mean blood lead levels. These findings were confirmed by a Norwegian study, where the occupational exposure of lead had been studied [101]. Furthermore, air pollution and its components are associated with preterm birth. Stieb et al. in their meta-analysis concluded that exposure to air pollution during the third trimester can lead to preterm birth. Nevertheless, this finding might be biased by the income or the socio-economic status of the study population, as Hispanic women are more likely to being exposed to air pollution than Black, Asian or White women. Phthalate exposure has been shown to be associated with preterm birth and specifically spontaneous preterm birth. Phthalate metabolites can act as endocrine disruptors and may lead to premature uterine contractions, resulting preterm labor and preterm birth [102-103]. The race with the highest exposure to phthalate metabolites exposure is the non-Hispanic Black race. Dichlorodiphenyltrichloroethane (DDT) an organochlorine used in agriculture and for malaria treatment has also been blamed for higher rates of preterm birth among women with higher DDT blood levels, with a dose-depended effect [104].

Padula et al. [105] studied the exposure level of women in Fresno County, California counting 19 environmental exposures in addition with the socioeconomic status of the population and they divided women in two sub-groups according to the exposure level (low or high exposure). They concluded that women who were included in the 'high exposure level' group had two times greater possibility to deliver prematurely compared to women in the 'low exposure' group. Concerning the drinking water contaminants, women with higher levels were more likely to experience preterm birth. More specifically, uranium and trichloroethylene were associated with early preterm birth while trihalomethans were a protective factor for preterm birth. Finally the scientists noticed that the relationship between pollution and preterm birth was stronger among areas with lower socio-economic status.

2.13. Nutritional Intake, Body Mass Index (BMI) and Gestational Weight Gain

Both excessive and insufficient gestational weight gain have been related to pregnancy complications, including preterm birth [106]. Women who were obese or over-weight before pregnancy (BMI >25 m/cm^2) should gain less weight during pregnancy, according to the updated IOM guidelines [107].However, less than 40% of pregnant women achieved gestational weight gain in line with the recommendations of IOM and 23% gained less weight than the recommended, while 37% gained more than the recommended weight. Women who gained less weight during pregnancy had 1.70 times higher risk for delivering prematurely, compared to women with normal weight gain. This association was stronger when compared to lower BMI; odds were 2.41 for underweight, 1.96 for normal weight, 1.55 for overweight and 1.20 for obese women. Surprisingly, gaining gestational weight over the IOM recommendations decreases the risk for preterm birth (OD: 0.77).

Regarding increased BMI as a single risk factor, several studies failed to prove a clear correlation with preterm birth [107-108].Usha Kiran et al. [109] concluded that women with increased BMI were more likely to have longer gestational periods, mainly due to hormonal disorders because of the excessive fat tissue. Smith et al. [110] in their study noticed that although women with increased BMI were less likely to deliver prematurely with spontaneous preterm labor, the possibility for iatrogenic preterm birth was higher.

The impact of nutritional factors on preterm birth has also been studied. A recent study from China suggested that decreased levels of vitamins B6, B12 and increased levels of homocysteine are considered risk factors for preterm birth [111]. Results from a recent study confirmed these findings and what they also showed was that women who take multi-vitamins pills and had adequate levels of these vitamins, showed decreased rates of preterm birth [112]. Omega-3 fatty acids also appear to have a protective role for preterm birth. Women who consumed adequate amounts of fish oils, fish and sea food, were shown to have 4-7 days longer pregnancy duration, while women who did not consume adequate amounts of these foods had 3.6 times higher risk for preterm birth [113-114].

2.14. Marital Status

Although in the modern western societies cohabitation is becoming more common and childbirth outside marriage is a common condition, according to Raatikainen et al. [115], "marriage still protects pregnancy." Several studies show that un-married women carry a higher risk for delivering prematurely compared to women who are married, and this correlation is stronger in countries where due to cultural or religious reasons childbearing outside marriage is less frequent [116]. Nevertheless, it is unclear whether marital status constitutes an independent risk factor for preterm birth, as in general unmarried women are more likely to have other risk factors for preterm birth such as: smoking before and during pregnancy, consumption of alcohol and drugs, adolescent pregnancy, unemployment and short interpregnancy intervals. Additionally, there is evidence suggesting that vaginal infections during pregnancy such as bacterial vaginosis is statistically more common in unmarried women. Also, epidemiologically unmarried pregnant women appear to be more vulnerable to emotional stress, they receive less social support and they adopt a riskier health behavior including dangerous sexual activity before and during pregnancy.

In Raatikainen's trial, unmarried women had increased incidence of preterm births than married women, with an odds ratio of 1.15 and absolute difference of 17.5%. Even after multivariate analysis, there was still statistically greater possibility for preterm birth. More specifically, for cohabiting women the OD remained 1.15, while for single mothers the possibility for preterm birth was increased, with an odds ratio of 1.29. Holt et al. [117] studied the change in marital status during pregnancy and they concluded that women who married before childbirth, achieved a reduction to the possibility of preterm birth.

2.15. Psychological Stress

Experiencing excessive psychological stress during pregnancy, such as stress fulevents (e.g., loss of a family member), perceived stress, anxiety, depressive symptoms or negative feelings and cumulative stress, has the potential to increase the risk of preterm birth [118]. In addition, pregnancy could be considered as a stressful event itself, as serious insecurities and concerns about childbirth and parenting are common in many women. Data from literature concerning stress and preterm birth show conflicting results; most studies run in the U.S. confirm the association of stress and preterm delivery, but the vast majority of European studies failed to confirm this relation, possibly due to the fact that they studied combination of outcomes, such as stress and SGA or depression and preterm birth and not the role of stress as an independent risk factor for preterm delivery [119]. McDonald et al. [119] in their survey confirmed that stress in general is a significant independent risk factor for late preterm birth (34-37 gestational weeks) with an OD of 1.79, while for early preterm birth this was not found to be statistically significant. After multi-variant analysis, women who were considered more optimistic or received social support were in less risk of delivering prematurely, while women with pessimistic attitude or not adequate social support had two-fold higher possibility for delivering prematurely. This was confirmed by a following study by Shapiro et al. [124]. Khashan et al. [120] proved that stressful events during pregnancy, namely major illness or death of a close-person increase preterm birth rates, even when they happened three months prior to conception. Women experiencing deaths in close family, delivered 4.6 weeks earlier compared to controls [121]. Additionally, pregnancy during war or natural disasters, e.g., catastrophic storms or earthquakes and run a higher risk of preterm delivery, specifically if pregnancy occurs during these events or even three months after, compared to pregnancies a year later [122,126-127]. However, Hedegaard et al. [123] claimed that stressful events by themselves have not the potential to lead to preterm delivery, but the way each woman experiences them might increase the possibilities for preterm birth. They also noticed that this perceived stress was statistically significant only if the stressful events were presented after the 30th gestational week. However, Zhu et al. [125] failed to confirm Hedegaard's finding, as they concluded that stressful life events could shorten gestational duration when experienced during the first or second trimester but not during the third.

Stress and preterm birth are related via neuroinflammatory, immune and neuroendocrine pathways [124]. The autonomic nervous system (ANS) is more active in women with preterm birth history, compared to women who delivered at term [122]. Dopaminergic activity and prefrontal function were measured via PET scan or functional MRI during stressful stimuli and it was found that they were significantly increased [127-128]. Furthermore, it is commonly accepted that infection is clearly associated with preterm birth. There is evidence proving that serum levels of proinflammatory cytokines of pregnant women experiencing stressful life events, are significantly increased, resulting to weakening of fetal membranes and ripening of the cervix [129]. Moreover, proinflammatory cytokines lead to production of prostaglandins which are molecular particles met just before the onset of labor and also during parturition. Despite the questions concerning stress and its role to preterm birth, the correlation with preterm birth, and increased levels of corticotrophin release hormone (CRH) is clear and it is proved that the Hypothalamus-Pituitary-Adrenal axis is the principal pathway linking stress and preterm birth [130]. Cortisol also increases prostaglandins' levels and decreases downregulation of prostaglandin metabolizing enzymes, accelerating paracrine and autocrine aspects of partirution [131].Finally, cortisol stimulates uterine contractions, premature myometrial activity and a cascade of events that lead to premature labor.

2.16. Employment

Employment's role on preterm birth prevalence has not been established, as studies regarding this issue could not draw a safe conclusion. According to Croteau et al. [132] standing for an excessive time in combination with occupational stress, increase the possibility of preterm birth. Other studies suggested that working during the night, or working for more than 42 hours per week and having a demanding physical job requiring more than 6 hours of standing, are associated with increased risk of preterm birth and more specifically with early preterm birth [133-135].Finally women who stated that their job is not satisfying, were more likely to deliver preterm compared to women who stated happy with their occupational environment.

2.17. Smoking

The connection of active smoking and preterm birth had been established since 1957 [136]. Nowadays, the adverse outcomes of smoking on health are very well-known, and healthcare policies have led to a reduction of smoking rates the last few years [137]. Recent data estimated that across Europe smoking rates range between 21% and 28% and about 10% of pregnant women continue to smoke during pregnancy. Smoking mainly leads to spontaneous preterm birth, while iatrogenic preterm birth is indicated because of secondary smoking consequences, such as placenta previa, placental abruption, or fetal growth restriction [140]. The correlation between smoking and preterm birth has a dose-depended effect: the more cigarettes one smokes, the greater the risk of delivering prematurely [138-139]. Additionally, according to Ko et al. [137] the risk for preterm birth was even greater when the mothers smoke more than 20 cigarettes per day. Shah and Bracken in their meta-analysis counted a 25% higher risk for preterm birth among women who continue smoking during pregnancy [141]. Among women smoking during pregnancy, the risk for delivering prematurely before the 32nd gestational week was 1.6-1.8 higher compared to nonsmokers, while the risk for late preterm birth was 1.3-1.4 higher [142].These numbers are in line with Ion's et al. [146] survey, who concluded that smoking during pregnancy is associated with a two-fold increase of preterm birth risk and they showed a 0.6 week reduction of gestational duration for smokers. Nevertheless, women who quit smoking from one pregnancy to the next, reduce their risk of preterm birth in the subsequent pregnancy, reaching the levels of nonsmokers [143]. A prospective study from New Zeeland showed that the risk of preterm birth among women who stop smoking before the 15th gestational week was equal to nonsmokers. The findings of the last two studies show that smoking effect on preterm birth is reversible, highlighting the need for proper counseling and encouraging pregnant women to quit smoking during pregnancy.

Despite the clear correlation between active smoking and preterm birth, in the current literature there are conflicting results concerning the association of environmental tobacco smoke exposure (ETSE) and preterm birth. According to Salmasi et al. [144], 22%-30% of pregnant women are exposed to tobacco smoke either at home or at work. Several meta-analyses failed to prove any statistically significant relation between ETSE and preterm birth. Ion et al. [146] noticed that exposed pregnant women showed a 0.19 week decrease on gestational duration, without any overall increased risk of preterm birth. Additionally, they calculated the exhaled carbon monoxide (eCO) levels during the first trimester of pregnancy and they found no association between eCO and any pregnancy complication. However, Kharrazi et al. [145] in their study concluded that passive smokers had 1.8 higher risk for delivering prematurely, compared to nonsmokers with a dose-response relation; the more the smokers at home, the higher the risk for preterm birth. Hyot el al also found that ETSE increases the risk for preterm birth [148]. They concluded that exposed mothers had a two-fold greater risk for preterm birth, compared to not exposed pregnant women.

2.18. Caffeine Consumption

The correlation between caffeine consumption during pregnancy and preterm birth is controversial. Studies that took place mainly in the 1990s suggested that caffeine had the potential to increase the risk for preterm birth with a dose-depended relation [149-150]. However, more recent surveys did not found an association between caffcine consumption and preterm birth [151-152].

2.19. Alcohol Consumption

The correlation between alcohol consumption during pregnancy and preterm birth is controversial, mainly due to the fact that the exact quantity of alcohol consumption is really difficult to be calculated. Additionally, different persons have different perceptions of what is defined as 'increased alcohol consumption'. The studies in the current literature give conflicting results concerning the relation between alcohol consumption and preterm birth. Landsberg et al. [153] concluded that even the consumption of two alcohol units per week during the third trimester of pregnancy has the potential to elevate preterm birth rates. In contrast, other scientists failed to prove any correlation between alcohol consumption and preterm birth, even when more than 21 alcohol units per week were consumed [154-156]. Interestingly, Pfinder et al. [157] claimed that alcohol consumption decreases preterm birth risk. Albertsen et al. [158] and Jaddoe et al. [159] came to an agreement with Landsber et al.

suggesting that the consumption of less than four alcohol units per week does not increase the possibilities for preterm birth. Albertsen et al. also calculated the threshold of consumption where the risk for delivering prematurely follows an upward trend and they estimated that drinking more than 7 alcohol units per week during pregnancy, could elevate preterm birth rates, while Parazzini et al. [160] calculated that the correlation between preterm birth and alcohol consumption, is starting to be statistically significant with the consumption of more than 3 alcohol units per week. Additionally, it is found that the association between alcohol consumption and preterm birth is stronger for the 'very preterm birth' (delivery before the 32nd gestational week).

2.20. Drugs

Drugs usage is one of the biggest social problems of the modern society, with the percentage of young adults and teenagers who use drugs, to follow an extreme upward trend. Additionally, 90% of the female users are in their reproductive age [161]. The association between drug's usage and preterm birth is controversial and it is unclear whether it is an independent risk factor for preterm birth, as women who use drugs are more likely to also have other risk factors, such as lower socio-economic status, smoking and co-morbidities [162].Slattery et al. [163] claimed that 25% of women taking drugs during pregnancy are going to deliver prematurely, while their risk is 3.45 times higher, compared to women who do not use drugs during pregnancy [164]. The opioid abuse during pregnancy increases the risk of preterm birth, with the responsible pathway remaining unclear. Concerning crack and cocaine usage during pregnancy they also increase the risk of preterm birth about 28.2% and 37% respectively [165-166]. Surprisingly the combined usage of cocaine and marijuana during pregnancy did not increase the risk of preterm birth [167-168], while other studies claimed that marijuana usage alone is associated with greater possibility of preterm birth [169].

CONCLUSION

Preterm birth is considered as a multi-factorial syndrome, and the origin of a great part of the causes of this syndrome are genetic, environmental and social, interacting dynamically, resulting to an even greater risk of preterm birth. The pathways leading a woman to deliver prematurely have not been well described yet, but the better known theories suggest that infections, utero-placental ischemia, stress or immune factors are the major causes resulting to preterm birth. Therefore, the exact mechanism responsible for preterm birth is very difficult to be defined, making even more important the identification of the epidemiological factors that may increase the risk for preterm birth. When these risk factors are well-known and well-understood, women at risk for delivering prematurely may be detected promptly, making possible the right guidance, even before conception, in order to decrease their risk, or give these women the opportunity to deliver in a safer environment. Additionally health care for these women could be personalized and some reversible risk factors such as smoking or alcohol consumption could be eliminated. Finally, the identification of the epidemiological factors responsible for preterm birth is the first step for better understanding of the mechanisms leading to preterm birth. In conclusion, as preterm birth is the major cause of neonatal mortality and morbidity it is of outmost importance for any obstetrician to have knowledge of the risk factors for preterm birth, to be able to detect these risk factors, to offer the best possible antenatal care to women at risk, to inform them properly and encourage them to alter some dangerous life-style habits, in order to reduce the possibilities and therefore the consequences of preterm birth.

REFERENCES

[1]   Chawanpaiboon S et al. Global, regional, and national estimates of levels of preterm birth in 2014: a systematic review and modelling analysis. *Lancet Glob Health* 2019; 7: e37–46.

[2] Leveno KJ, Cunninghan FG, Gant NF, Alexander JM, Bloom SL, Casey BM, Sheffield JS, Vost NP. Part V: Obstetrical complications due to pregnancy: *"Williams manual of obstetrics,"* 21st edition. McGraw-Hill Company, 2003; 397-414.

[3] Lumley J. Defining the problem: the epidemiology of preterm birth. *BJOG.* 2003 Apr;110 Suppl 20:3-7.

[4] Haram K, Mortensen JH, Wollen AL. Preterm delivery: an overview. *Acta Obstet Gynecol Scand.* 2003 Aug;82(8):687-704.

[5] Eliyahu S, Weiner E, Nachum Z, Shalev E. Epidemiologic risk factors for Preterm Delivery. *IMAJ* 2002;4:1115-1117.

[6] Blencowe H, Cousens S, Chou D, Oestergaard M, Say L, Moller AB, Kinney M, Lawn J; Born Too Soon Preterm Birth Action Group. Born too soon: the global epidemiology of 15 million preterm births. *Reprod Health.* 2013;10 Suppl 1:S2. doi:10.1186/1742-4755-10-S1-S2. Epub 2013 Nov 15.

[7] Goldenberg RL, Culhane JF, Iams JD, Romero R. Epidemiology and causes of preterm birth. *Lancet.* 2008 Jan 5;371(9606):75-84. doi:10.1016/S0140-6736(08)60074-4.

[8] Howson CP, Kinney MV, McDougall L, Lawn JE; Born Too Soon Preterm Birth Action Group. Born Too Soon: Preterm birth matters. *Reproductive Health* 2013, 10(Suppl 1):S1.

[9] Liu L, Johnson HL, Cousens S, Perin J, Scott S, Lawn JE, Rudan I, Campbell H, Cibulskis R, Li M, et al. Global, regional, and national causes of child mortality: an updated systematic analysis for 2010 with time trends since 2000. *Lancet* 2012, 379:2151-2161.

[10] Blencowe H, Lee AC, Cousens S, Bahalim A, Narwal R, Zhong N, Chou D, Say L, Modi N, Katz J, et al. Preterm birth associated impairment estimates at regional and global level for 2010. *Pediatric Research.*

[11] Motquin JM. Classification and heterogenity of preterm birth. *BJOG* 2003;110(20):30-33.

[12] Phillips C, Velji Z, Hanly C, Metcalfe A. Risk of recurrent spontaneous preterm birth: a systematic review and meta-analysis.

BMJ Open. 2017 Jul 5;7(6):e015402. doi:10.1136/bmjopen-2016-015402.

[13] Phillips C, Velji Z, Hanly C, et al. Risk of recurrent spontaneous preterm birth: a systematic review and meta-analysis. *BMJ Open* 2017;7:e015402. doi:10.1136/bmjopen-2016-015402.

[14] Kazemier BM, Buijs PE, Mignini L, et al. Impact of obstetric history on the risk of spontaneous preterm birth in singleton and multiple pregnancies: a systematic review. *BJOG* 2014;121:1197–208. discussion 209.

[15] Shapiro GD, Fraser WD, Frasch MG, et al. Psychosocial stress in pregnancy and preterm birth: associations and mechanisms. *J Perinat Med* 2013;41:631–45.

[16] Loomans EM, van Dijk AE, Vrijkotte TG, et al. Psychosocial stress during pregnancy is related to adverse birth outcomes: results from alarge multi-ethnic community-based birth cohort. *Eur J Public Health* 2013;23:485–91.

[17] Ananth CV, Vintzileos AM. Epidemiology of preterm birth and its clinical subtypes. *J Matern Fetal Neonatal Med* 2006;19:773–82.

[18] Yang J, Baer RJ, Berghella V, Chambers C, Chung P, Coker T, Currier RJ, Druzin ML, Kuppermann M, Muglia LJ, Norton ME, Rand L, Ryckman K, Shaw GM, Stevenson D, Jelliffe-Pawlowski LL. Recurrence of Preterm Birth and Early Term Birth. *Obstet Gynecol.* 2016 Aug;128(2):364-72. doi:10.1097/AOG.0000000000001506.

[19] Ward K. Genetic factors in preterm birth. *BJOG.* 2003 Apr;110 Suppl 20:117.

[20] Haram K, Mortensen JH, Wollen AL. Preterm delivery: an overview. *Acta Obstet Gynecol Scand.*2003 Aug;82(8):687-704.

[21] Fox NS, Roman AS, Stern EM, Gerber RS, Saltzman DH, Rebarber A. Type of congenital uterine anomaly and adverse pregnancy outcomes. *J Matern Fetal Neonatal Med,* 2014; 27(9): 949–953.

[22] Chan YY, Jayaprakasan K, Tan A, et al. Reproductive outcomes in women with congenital uterine anomalies: a systematic review. *Ultrasound Obstet Gynecol* 2011;38:371–82.

[23] Parazzini F, Tozzi L, Bianchi S, Pregnancy outcome and uterine fibroids, *Best Practice & Research Clinical Obstetrics &Gynaecology* (2015), doi: 10.1016/j.bpobgyn.2015.11.017.

[24] Klatsky PC, Tran ND, Caughey AB, et al. Fibroids and reproductive outcomes: a systematic literature review from conception to delivery. *Am J Obstet Gynecol.* 2008;198:357-366.

[25] Chen YH, Lin HC, Chen SF, et al. Increased risk of preterm births among women with uterine leiomyoma: a nationwide population-based study. *Hum Reprod.* 2009;24:3049-3056.

[26] Lai J, Caughey AB, Qidwai GI, et al. Neonatal outcomes in women with sonographically identified uterine leiomyomata. *J Matern Fetal Neonatal Med.* 2012;25:710-713.

[27] Navid S, Arshad S, Quratul A, et al. Impact of leiomyoma in pregnancy. *J Ayub Med Coll Abbottabad.* 2012;24:90-92.

[28] Shavell VI, Thakur M, Sawant A, et al. Adverse obstetric outcomes associated with sonographically identified large uterine fibroids. *Fertil Steril.* 2012;97:107-110.

[29] Deveer M, Deveer R, Engin-Ustun Y, et al. Comparison of pregnancy outcomes in different localizations of uterine fibroids. *Clin Exp Obstet Gynecol.* 2012;39:516-518.

[30] Lam SJ, Best S & Kumar S. The impact of fibroid characteristics on pregnancy outcome. *Am J Obstet Gynecol.* 2014;211:395 e391-395.

[31] Ezzedine Dima, Norwitz Errol. Are Women With Uterine Fibroids at Increased Risk for Adverse Pregnancy Outcome? *Clinical Obstetrics and Gynecology.* Volume 59, Number 1, 119–127.

[32] Norman J and Greer I. Preterm Labour: managing risk in clinical practice. Chapter 1. *The epidemiology of preterm labour and delivery.* Cambridge University Press pp. 6.

[33] Smith GC, Pell JP, Dobbie R. Interpregnancy interval and risk of preterm birth and neonatal death: retrospective cohort study. *BMJ.* 2003 Aug 9;327(7410):313.

[34] Winkvist, A., Rasmussen, K. M., & Habicht, J. P. (1992). A new definition of maternal depletion syndrome. *American Journal of Public Health, 82*(5), 691–694.

[35] Lin, J, Liu, H, Wu, DD, Hu, HT, Wang, HH, Zhou, CL, Liu, XM, Chen, XJ, Sheng, JZ, and Huang, HF. (2019). Long interpregnancy interval and adverse perinatal outcomes: A retrospective cohort study. *Sci China Life Sci* 6 https://doi.org/10.1007/s11427-018-9593-8.

[36] Hegelund ER, Urhoj SK, Andersen AN, Mortensen LH. Interpregnancy Interval and Risk of Adverse Pregnancy Outcomes: A Register-Based Study of 328,577 Pregnancies in Denmark 1994-2010. *Matern Child Health J.* 2018 Jul;22(7):1008-1015. doi:10.1007/s10995-018-2480-7.

[37] Zhu, BP, Rolfs, RT, Nangle, BE, & Horan, JM. (1999). Effect of the interval between pregnancies on perinatal outcomes. *New England Journal of Medicine, 340*(8), 589–594.

[38] Hsieh TT, Chen SF, Shau WY, Hsieh CC, Hsu JJ, Hung TH. The impact of interpregnancy interval and previous preterm birth on the subsequent risk of preterm birth. *J Soc Gynecol Investig.* 2005 Apr;12(3):202-7.

[39] Hanley, GE, Hutcheon, JA, Kinniburgh, BA, and Lee, L. (2017). Interpregnancy interval and adverse pregnancy outcomes. *Obstetrics Gynecol* 129, 408–415.

[40] Conde-Agudelo A, Rosas-Bermúdez A, Kafury-Goeta AC. Birth spacing and risk of adverse perinatal outcomes: a meta-analysis. *JAMA* 2006;295(15):1809–1823.

[41] Owen J, Yost N, Berghella V, et al. Mid-trimester endovaginal sonography in women at high risk for spontaneous preterm birth. *JAMA* 2001;286:1340e8.

[42] Miller ES, Tita AT, Grobman WA. Second-trimester cervical length screening among asymptomatic women: an evaluation of risk-based strategies. *Obstet Gynecol* 2015;126:61e6.

[43] Ville y, Rozenberg P, Predictors of Preterm Birth, Best Practice & Research. *Clinical Obstetrics & Gynaecology* (2018), doi: 10.1016/j.bpobgyn.2018.05.002.

[44] Kuoppala T, Saarikoski S. Pregnancy and delivery after cone biopsy of the cervix. *Arch Gynecol.* 1986;237(3):149-54.

[45] Larsson G, Grundsell H, Gullberg B, Svennerud S. Outcome of pregnancy after conization. *Acta Obstet Gynecol Scand.* 1982;61(5):461-6.

[46] Moinian M, Andersch B. Does cervix conization increase the risk of complications in subsequent pregnancies? *Acta Obstet Gynecol Scand.* 1982;61(2):101-3.

[47] Jakobsson M, Gissler M, Sainio S, Paavonen J, Tapper AM. Preterm delivery after surgical treatment for cervical intraepithelial neoplasia. *Obstet Gynecol* 2007 Feb;109(2 Pt 1):309-13.

[48] Kyrgiou M, Koliopoulos G, Martin-Hirsch P, Arbyn M, Prendiville W, Paraskevaidis E. Obstetric outcomes after conservative treatment for intraepithelial or early invasive cervical lesions: systematic review and meta-analysis. *Lancet.* 2006 Feb 11;367(9509):489-98.

[49] Kyrgiou M, Athanasiou A, Kalliala IEJ, Paraskevaidi M, Mitra A, Martin-Hirsch PPL, Arbyn M, Bennett P, Paraskevaidis E. Obstetric outcomes after conservative treatment for cervical intraepithelial lesions and early invasive disease. *Cochrane Database of Systematic Reviews* 2017, Issue 11. Art. No.: CD012847. doi: 10.1002/ 14651858.CD01284.

[50] KyrgiouM, et al. Adverse obstetric outcomes after local treatment for cervical preinvasive and early invasive disease according to cone depth: systematic review and meta-analysis.*BMJ*2016;354:i3633. http://dx.doi.org/10.1136/bmj.i3633.

[51] McCarthy FP, Khashan AS, North RA, Rahma MB, Walker JJ, Baker PN, Dekker G, Poston L, McCowan LM, O'Donoghue K, Kenny LC; SCOPE Consortium. Pregnancy loss managed by cervical dilatation and curettage increases the risk of spontaneous preterm birth. *Hum Reprod.* 2013 Dec;28(12):3197-206. doi:10.1093/ humrep/det332. Epub 2013 Sep 19.

[52] Virk J, Zhang J, Olsen J. Medical abortion and the risk of subsequent adverse pregnancy outcomes. *N Engl J Med* 2007;357:648–653.

[53] Oliver-Williams C, Fleming M, Wood AM, Smith G. Previous miscarriage and the subsequent risk of preterm birth in Scotland,

1980-2008: a historical cohort study. *BJOG.* 2015 Oct;122(11):1525-34. doi:10.1111/1471-0528.13276. Epub 2015 Jan 28.

[54] Carolan M. Maternal age >45 years and maternal and perinatal outcomes: A review of the evidence. *Midwifery* 29 (2013) 479–489.

[55] Lawlor D, Monrtensen L, Nybo Antersen AM. Mechanisms underlying the associations of maternal age with adverse perinatal outcomes: a sibling study of 264 695 Danish women and their firstborn offspring *International Journal of Epidemiology* 2011;40:1205–1214 doi:10.1093/ije/dyr084.

[56] Fuchs F, Monet B, Ducruet T, Chaillet N, Audibert F. (2018) Effect of maternal age on the risk of preterm birth: A large cohort study. *PLoS ONE* 13(1): e0191002. https://doi.org/10.1371/journal.pone.0191002.

[57] Goisis A, Remes H, Barclay K, Martikainen P, Myrskylä M. Advanced Maternal Age and the Risk of Low Birth Weight and Preterm Delivery: a Within-Family Analysis Using Finnish Population Registers. *Am J Epidemiol.* 2017 Dec 1;186(11):1219-1226. doi:10.1093/aje/kwx177.

[58] Khalil A, Syngelaki A, Maiz N, Zinevich Y, Nicolaides KH. Maternal age and adverse pregnancy outcome: a cohort study. *Ultrasound Obstet Gynecol.* 2013 Dec;42(6):634-43. doi:10.1002/uog.12494.

[59] Azevedo WF, Diniz MB, Fonseca ES, Azevedo LM, Evangelista CB. Complications in adolescent pregnancy: systematic review of the literature. 2015 Oct-Dec;13(4):618-26. doi:10.1590/S1679-45082015RW3127. Epub 2015 Jun 9.

[60] Stewart CP, Katz J, Khatry SK, LeClerq SC, Shrestha SR, West KP Jr, et al. Preterm delivery but not intrauterine growth retardation is associated with young maternal age among primiparae in rural Nepal. *Matern Child Nutr.* 2007;3(3):174-85.

[61] Kongnyuy EJ, Nana PN, Fomulu N, Wiysonge SC, Kouam L, Doh AS. Adverse perinatal outcomes of adolescent pregnancies in Cameroon. *Matern Child Health J.* 2008;12(2):149-54.

[62] Leftwich HK, Alves MV. Adolescent Pregnancy. *Pediatr Clin North Am.* 2017 Apr;64(2):381-388. doi:10.1016/j.pcl.2016.11.007. Epub 2017 Jan 3.

[63] KushnirVA,Barad DH,Albertini DF,Darmon SK. Systematic review of world wide trends in assisted reproductive technology 2004-2013. *Reprod Biol Endocrinol.*2017 Jan 10;15(1):6. doi:10.1186/s12958-016-0225-2.

[64] Helmerhorst FM, Perquin DA, Donker D, Keirse MJ. Perinatal outcome of singletons and twins after assisted conception: a systematic review of controlled studies. *BMJ.* 2004 Jan 31;328(7434):261.

[65] Filicori M, Cognigni GE, Gamberini E, Troilo E, Parmegiani L, Bernardi S. Impact of medically assisted fertility on preterm birth. *BJOG.*2005 Mar;112 Suppl 1:113-7.

[66] Perri T, Chen R, Yoeli R, et al. Are singleton assisted reproductive technology pregnancies at risk of prematurity? *J Assist Reprod Genet* 2001; 18: 245– 249. doi: 10.1023/A:1016614217411.

[67] Henriksen TB, Baird DD, Olsen J, Hedegaard M, Secher NJ, Wilcox AJ. Time to pregnancy and preterm delivery. *Obstet Gynecol* 1997; 89: 594– 599. doi: 10.1016/S0029-7844(97)00045-8.

[68] Luke B, Pregnancy and Birth Outcomes in Couples with Infertility With and Without Assisted Reproductive Technology: With an Emphasis on US Population-Based Studies, *American Journal of Obstetrics and Gynecology* (2017), doi: 10.1016/j.ajog.2017.03.012.

[69] Wang JX, Norman RJ, Kristiansson P. The eect of various infertility treatments on the risk of preterm birth. *Hum Reprod* 2002; 17: 945– 949. doi: 10.1093/humrep/17.4.945.

[70] Fuchs F, Senat MV. Multiple gestations and preterm birth. *Semin Fetal Neonatal Med.* 2016 Apr;21(2):113-20. doi:10.1016/j.siny. 2015.12.010. Epub 2016 Jan 13.

[71] Slattery MM, Morrison JJ. Preterm Delivery. *Lancet* 2002;360:148997.

[72] Martin JA, Hamilton BE, Osterman MJK, Curtin SC, Mathews TJ. National vital statistics reports. *Births: final data for 2013.* 2015.

[73] Conde-Agudelo A, Romero R, Hassan SS, Yeo L. Transvaginal sonographic cervical length for the prediction of spontaneous preterm birth in twin pregnancies: a systematic review and metaanalysis. *Am J Obstet Gynecol* 2010;203. 128 e1e12.

[74] Penava D, Natale R. An association of chorionicity with preterm twin birth. *J Obstet Gynaecol Can.* 2004 Jun;26(6):571-4.

[75] Breathnach FM, McAuliffe FM, Geary M, Daly S, Higgins JR, Dornan J, et al. Optimum timing for planned delivery of uncomplicated monochorionic and dichorionic twin pregnancies. *Obstet Gynecol* 2012;119(1):50e9.

[76] Joseph KS, Marcoux S, Ohlsson A, Kramer MS, Allen AC, Liu S, Wu Wen S, Demissie K, Sauve R, Liston R; Fetal and Infant Health Study Group of the Canadian Perinatal Surveillance System. Preterm birth, stillbirth and infant mortality among triplet births in Canada, 1985-96. *Paediatr Perinat Epidemiol.* 2002 Apr;16(2):141-8.

[77] Stock S, Norman J. Preterm and term labour in multiple pregnancies. *Semin Fetal Neonatal Med* 2010;15:336e41.

[78] Tough SC, Newburn-Cook C, Johnston DW, Svenson LW, Rose S, Belik J. Delayed childbearing and its impact on population rate changes in lower birth weight, multiple birth, and preterm delivery. *Pediatrics.* 2002 Mar;109(3):399-403.

[79] Hall MH (1985) Incidence and distribution of preterm labour. In RW Beard and F Sharp eds., *Preterm Labour and its consequences.* London: pp.5-13.

[80] Kumari AS, Badrinath P. Extreme grand multiparity: is it an obstetric risk factor? *Eur J Obstet Gynecol Reprod Biol.* 2002 Feb 10;101(1):22-5.

[81] Byrne B, Morrison JJ. Preterm birth. *Clin Evid.* 2002 Dec;(8):1491-505.

[82] Hegelund ER, Poulsen GJ, Mortensen LH. Educational Attainment and Pregnancy Outcomes: A Danish Register-Based Study of the Influence of Childhood Social Disadvantage on Later Socioeconomic Disparities in Induced Abortion, Spontaneous

Abortion, Stillbirth and PretermDelivery. *Matern Child Health J.*2019 Jun;23(6):839-846. doi:10.1007/s10995-018-02704-1.

[83] Burris HH, Hacker MR. Birth outcome racial disparities: A result of intersecting social and environmental factors. *Semin Perinatol.*2017 Oct;41(6):360-366. doi:10.1053/j.semperi.2017.07.002. Epub 2017 Aug 18.

[84] Earnings and unemployment rates by educational attainment. *Bureau of Labor Statistics.* https://www.bls.gov/emp/ep_table_001.htm. Accessed January 24, 2017.

[85] Manuck TA. Racial and ethnic differences in preterm birth: A complex, multifactorial problem. *Semin Perinatol.*2017 Dec;41(8):511-518. doi: 10.1053/j.semperi.2017.08.010. Epub 2017 Sep 21.

[86] Schaaf JM, Liem SM, Mol BW, Abu-Hanna A, Ravelli AC. Ethnic and racial disparities in the risk of preterm birth: a systematic review and meta-analysis. *Am J Perinatol.* 2013;30: 433–450.

[87] Plunkett J, Borecki I, Morgan T, Stamilio D, Muglia LJ. Population-based estimate of sibling risk for preterm birth, preterm premature rupture of membranes, placental abruption and pre-eclampsia. *BMC Genet.* 2008;9:44.

[88] Frey HA, Stout MJ, Pearson LN, et al. Genetic variation associated with preterm birth in African-American women. *Am J Obstet Gynecol.* 2016;215:235 e1-8.

[89] Cruickshank MN, Oshlack A, Theda C, et al. Analysis of epigenetic changes in survivors of preterm birth reveals the effect of gestational age and evidence for a long term legacy. *Genome Med.* 2013;5:96.

[90] Parets SE, Conneely KN, Kilaru V, et al. Fetal DNA methylation associates with early spontaneous preterm birth and gestational age. *PLoS One.* 2013;8:e67489.

[91] Jones CW, Gambala C, Esteves KC, et al. Differences in placental telomere length suggest a link between racial disparities in birth outcomes and cellular aging. *Am J Obstet Gynecol.* 2017;216:294 [e1–e8].

[92] Khalil A, Rezende J, Akolekar R, Syngelaki A, Nicolaides KH. Maternal racial origin and adverse pregnancy outcome: a cohort study. *Ultrasound Obstet Gynecol.* 2013 Mar;41(3):278-85. doi: 10.1002/uog.12313.

[93] Gurer-Orhan H, Sabir HU, Ozgunes H. Correlation between clinical indicators of lead poisoning and oxidative stress parameters in controls and lead-exposed workers. *Toxicology.* 2004;195(2–3):147–154.

[94] Kelly FJ. Oxidative stress: its role in air pollution and adverse health effects. *Occup Environ Med.* 2003;60(8):612–616.

[95] Ferguson KK, McElrath TF, Chen YH, Mukherjee B, Meeker JD. Urinary phthalate metabolites and biomarkers of oxidative stress in pregnant women: a repeated measures analysis. *Environ Health Perspect.* 2015;123(3):210–216.

[96] Pope CA 3rd, Hansen ML, Long RW, et al. Ambient particulate air pollution, heart rate variability, and blood markers of inflammation in a panel of elderly subjects. *Environ Health Perspect.* 2004;112(3):339–345.

[97] Ferguson KK, Loch-Caruso R, Meeker JD. Urinary phthalate metabolites in relation to biomarkers of inflammation and oxidative stress: NHANES 1999–2006. *Environ Res.* 2011;111(5): 718–726.

[98] Williams DR, Collins C. Racial residential segregation: a fundamental cause of racial disparities in health. *Public Health Rep.* 2001;116(5):404–416.

[99] Andrews KW, Savitz DA, Hertz-Picciotto I. Prenatal lead exposure in relation to gestational age and birth weight: a review of epidemiologic studies. *Am J Ind Med.* 1994;26(1): 13–32.

[100] Irgens A, Kruger K, Skorve AH, Irgens LM. Reproductive outcome in offspring of parents occupationally exposed to lead in Norway. *Am J Ind Med.* 1998;34(5):431–437.

[101] Ferguson KK, McElrath TF, Meeker JD. Environmental phthalate exposure and preterm birth. *JAMA Pediatr.* 2014;168(1): 61–67. 43.

[102] Meeker JD, Hu H, Cantonwine DE, et al. Urinary phthalate metabolites in relation to preterm birth in Mexico city. *Environ Health Perspect.* 2009;117(10):1587–1592.

[103] Kelly K. Ferguson, Marie S. O'Neill & John D. Meeker (2013): Environmental Contaminant Exposures and Preterm Birth: A Comprehensive Review, *Journal of Toxicology and Environmental Health, Part B: Critical Reviews*, 16:2, 69-11.

[104] Padula AM, Huang H, Baer RJ, August LM, Jankowska MM, Jellife-Pawlowski LL, Sirota M, Woodruff TJ. Environmental pollution and social factors as contributors to preterm birth in Fresno County. *Environ Health.* 2018 Aug 29;17(1):70. doi:10.1186/s12940-018-0414-x.

[105] Goldstein RF, Abell SK, Ranasinha S, Misso M, Boyle JA, Black MH, Li N, Hu G, Corrado F, Rode L, Kim YJ, Haugen M, Song WO, Kim MH, Bogaerts A, Devlieger R, Chung JH, Teede HJ. Association of Gestational Weight Gain with Maternal and Infant Outcomes: A Systematic Review and Meta-analysis. *JAMA.* 2017 Jun 6;317(21):2207-2225. doi: 10.1001/jama.2017.3635.

[106] Rasmussen K, Yaktine AL, eds; Institute of Medicine; National Research Council. *Weight Gain During Pregnancy: Reexamining the Guidelines.* Washington, DC: National Academies Press; 2009.

[107] Usha Kiran TS, Hemmadi S, Bethel J, Evans J. Outcome of pregnancy in a woman with an increased body mass index. *BJOG.* 2005 Jun;112(6):768-72.

[108] Kramer MS, Lydon J, Séguin L, Goulet L, Kahn SR, McNamara H, Genest J, Dassa C, Chen MF, Sharma S, Meaney MJ, Thomson S, Van Uum S, Koren G, Dahhou M, Lamoureux J, Platt RW. Stress pathways to spontaneous preterm birth: the role of stressors, psychological distress, and stress hormones. *Am J Epidemiol.* 2009 Jun 1;169(11):1319-26.

[109] Smith GC, Shah I, Pell JP, Crossley JA, Dobbie R. Maternal obesity in early pregnancy and risk of spontaneous and elective preterm deliveries: a retrospective cohort study. *Am J Public Health.* 2007 Jan;97(1):157-62.

[110] Ronnenberg AG, Goldman MB, Chen D, Aitken IW, Willett WC, Selhub J, Xu X. Preconception homocysteine and B vitamin status and birth outcomes in Chinese women. *Am J Clin Nutr.* 2002 Dec;76(6):1385-91.

[111] Vahratian A, Siega-Riz AM, Savitz DA, Thorp JM Jr. Multivitamin use and the risk of preterm birth. *Am J Epidemiol.* 2004 Nov 1;160(9):886-92.

[112] Olsen SF, Secher NJ. Low consumption of seafood in early pregnancy as a risk factor for preterm delivery: prospective cohort study. *BMJ.* 2002 Feb 23;324(7335):447.

[113] Facchinetti F, Fazzio M, Venturini P. Polyunsaturated fatty acids and risk of preterm delivery. *Eur Rev Med Pharmacol Sci.* 2005 Jan-Feb;9(1):41-8.

[114] Raatikainen K,Heiskanen N,Heinonen S. Marriage still protects pregnancy. *BJOG.*2005 Oct;112(10):1411-6.

[115] Zeitlin JA, Saurel-Cubizolles MJ, Ancel PY, EUROPOP Group. Marital status, cohabitation, and risk of preterm birth in Europe: where births outside marriage are common and uncommon. *Paediatr Perinat Epidemiol* 2002;16(2):124 – 130.

[116] Holt VL, Danoff NL, Mueller BA, Swanson MW. The association of change in maternal marital status between births and adverse pregnancy outcomes in the second birth.*Paediatr Perinat Epidemiol.* 1997 Jan;11 Suppl 1:31-40.

[117] Orr ST, Reiter JP, Blazer DG, James SA (2007) Maternal prenatal pregnancy-related anxiety and spontaneous preterm birth in Baltimore, Maryland. *Psychosom Med* 69(6):566–570.

[118] McDonald SW, Kingston D, Bayrampour H, Dolan SM, Tough SC. Cumulative psychosocial stress, coping resources, and preterm birth. *Arch Womens Ment Health.* 2014 Dec;17(6):559-68. doi:10.1007/s00737-014-0436-5. Epub 2014 Jun 20.

[119] Khashan AS, McNamee R, Abel KM, Mortensen PB, Kenny LC, Pedersen MG, Webb RT, Baker PN. Rates of preterm birth following antenatal maternal exposure to severe life events: a

population-based cohort study. *Hum Reprod.* 2009 Feb;24(2):429-37.

[120] Hedegaard M, Henriksen TB, Secher NJ, Hatch MC, Sabroe S. Do stressful life events affect duration of gestation and risk of preterm delivery? *Epidemiology*.1996 Jul;7(4):339-45.

[121] Hogan VK, Richardson JL, Ferre CD, Durant T, Boisseau M. A public health framework for addressing black and white disparities in preterm delivery. *J Am Med Womens Assoc.* 2001;56:177-180.

[122] Omer H, Everly GS Jr. Psychological factors in preterm labor: critical review and theoretical synthesis. *Am J Psychiatry*.1988 Dec;145(12):1507-13.

[123] Shapiro G, Fraser W, Frasch M, Seguin J. Psychosocial stress in pregnancy and preterm birth: associations and mechanisms. *J. Perinat. Med.* 2013; 41(6): 631–645.

[124] Zhu P, Tao F, Hao J, Sun Y, Jiang X. Prenatal life events stress: implications for preterm birth and infant birthweight. *Am J Obstet Gynecol.* 2010;203:34 e1–8.

[125] Glynn LM, Wadhwa PD, Dunkel-Schetter C, Chicz-Demet A, Sandman CA. When stress happens matters: effects of earthquake timing on stress responsivity in pregnancy. *Am J Obstet Gynecol.* 2001;184:637–42.

[126] Dancause KN, Laplante DP, Oremus C, Fraser S, Brunet A, King S. Disaster-related prenatal maternal stress influences birth outcomes: Project Ice Storm. *Early Hum Dev.* 2011;87:813–20.

[127] Lataster J, Collip D, Ceccarini J, Haas D, Booij L, van Os J, et al. Psychosocial stress is associated with in vivo dopamine release in human ventromedial prefrontal cortex: a positron emission tomography study using [(1)(8)F]fallypride. *Neuroimage.* 2011;58:1081–9.

[128] Liston C, McEwen BS, Casey BJ. Psychosocial stress reversibly disrupts prefrontal processing and attentional control. *Proc Natl Acad Sci USA.* 2009;106:912–7.

[129] Christian LM. Psychoneuroimmunology in pregnancy: Immune pathways linking stress with maternal health, adverse birth

outcomes, and fetal development. *Neurosci Biobehav Rev.* 2012;36:350–61.

[130] Dunkel Schetter C. Psychological science on pregnancy: stress processes, biopsychosocial models, and emerging research issues. *Annu Rev Psychol.* 2011;62:531–58.

[131] Challis JR, Sloboda D, Matthews SG, Holloway A, Alfaidy N, Patel FA, et al. The fetal placental hypothalamic-pituitaryadrenal (HPA) axis, parturition and post natal health. *Mol Cell Endocrinol.* 2001;185:135–44.

[132] Croteau A, Marcoux S, Brisson C. Work activity in pregnancy, preventive measures, and the risk of preterm delivery.*Am J Epidemiol.* 2007 Oct 15;166(8):951-65.

[133] Pompeii LA, Savitz DA, Evenson KR, Rogers B, McMahon M. Physical exertion at work and the risk of preterm delivery and small-for-gestational-age birth. *Obstet Gynecol.* 2005 Dec;106(6):1279-88.

[134] Lawson CC, Whelan EA, Hibert EN, Grajewski B, Spiegelman D, Rich-Edwards JW. Occupational factors and risk of preterm birth in nurses. *Am J Obstet Gynecol.*2009 Jan;200(1):51.e1-8.

[135] Saurel-Cubizolles MJ, Zeitlin J, Lelong N, Papiernik E, Di Renzo GC, Bréart G; Europop Group. Employment, working conditions, and preterm birth: results from the Europop case-control survey. *J Epidemiol Community Health.* 2004 May;58(5):395-401.

[136] Simpson WJ, Linda L. A preliminary report on cigarette smoking and the incidence of prematurity. *Am J Obstet Gynecol.* 1957; 73(4):807-815.

[137] World Health Organisation. Report on the Global Tobacco Epidemic - the MPOWER Package. Geneva: World Health Organisation; 2008.

[138] Ko TJ, Tsai LY, Chu LC, Yeh SJ, Leung C, Chen CY, Chou HC, Tsao PN, Chen PC, Hsieh WS. Parental smoking during pregnancy and its association with lowbirth weight, small for gestational age, and preterm birth off spring: a birth cohort study. *Pediatr Neonatol.*2014 Feb;55(1):20-7. doi:10.1016/j.pedneo.2013.05.005. Epub 2013 Jul 12.

[139] Ion R, Bernal AL. Smoking and Preterm Birth. *Reprod Sci.* 2015 Aug;22(8):918-26. doi:10.1177/1933719114556486. Epub 2014 Nov 12.

[140] Castles A, Adams EK, Melvin CL, Kelsch C, Boulton ML. Effects of smoking during pregnancy. Five meta-analyses. *Am J Prev Med.* 1999;16(3):208-215.

[141] Shah NR, Bracken MB. A systematic review and meta-analysis of prospective studies on the association between maternal cigarette smoking and preterm delivery. *Am J Obstet Gynecol.* 2000; 182(2):465-472.

[142] Gardosi J, Francis A. Early pregnancy predictors of preterm birth: the role of a prolonged menstruation–conception interval. *Br J Obstet Gynaecol* 2000;107: 228–237.

[143] Cnattingius S, Granath F, Petersson G, Harlow BL. The influence of gestational age and smoking habits on the risk of subsequent preterm deliveries. *N Engl J Med.* 1999;341(13):943-948.

[144] Salmasi G, Grady R, Jones J, McDonald SD, Group KS. Environmental tobacco smoke exposure and perinatal outcomes: systematic review and meta-analyses. *Acta Obstet Gynecol Scand.* 2010;89(4):423-441.

[145] Kharrazi M, DeLorenze GN, Kaufman FL, et al. Environmental tobacco smoke and pregnancy outcome. *Epidemiology.* 2004; 15(6):660-670.

[146] Ion RC, Wills AK, Bernal AL. Environmental Tobacco Smoke Exposure in Pregnancy is Associated with Earlier Delivery and Reduced Birth Weight. *Reprod Sci.*2015 Dec;22(12):1603-11. doi:10.1177/1933719115612135. Epub 2015 Oct 27.

[147] Fantuzzi G, Aggazzotti G, Righi E, et al. Preterm delivery and exposure to active and passive smoking during pregnancy: a case-control study from Italy. *Paediatr Perinat Epidemiol.* 2007;21(3):194-200.

[148] Hoyt AT, Canfield MA, Romitti PA, Botto LD, Anderka MT, Krikov SV, Feldkamp ML. Does Maternal Exposure to Secondhand Tobacco Smoke During Pregnancy Increase the Risk for Pretermor

Small-for-Gestational Age Birth? *Matern Child Health J.* 2018 Oct;22(10):1418-1429.

[149] Williams MA, Mittendorf R, Stubblefield PG, Lieberman E, Schoenbaum SC, Monson RR. Cigarettes, coffee, and preterm premature rupture of the membranes. *Am J Epidemiol.* 1992 Apr 15;135(8):895-903.

[150] Eskenazi B, Stapleton AL, Kharrazi M, Chee WY. Associations between maternal decaffeinated and caffeinated coffee consumption and fetal growth and gestational duration. *Epidemiology.* 1999 May;10(3):242-9.

[151] Vitti FP, Grandi C, Cavalli RC, Simões VMF, Batista RFL, Cardoso VC. Association between Caffeine Consumption in Pregnancy and Low Birth Weight and Preterm Birth in the birth Cohort of Ribeirão Preto. *Rev Bras Ginecol Obstet.* 2018 Dec;40(12):749-756. doi:10.1055/s-0038-1675806. Epub 2018 Dec 7.

[152] Bech BH, Obel C, Henriksen TB, Olsen J. Effect of reducing caffeine intake on birth weight and length of gestation: randomised controlled trial. *BMJ.* 2007 Feb 24;334(7590):409.

[153] Lundsberg LS, Bracken MB, Saftlas AF. Low-to-moderate gestational alcohol use and intrauterine growth retardation, low birthweight, and preterm delivery. *Ann Epidemiol.* 1997 Oct;7(7):498-50.

[154] Kesmodel U, Olsen SF, Secher NJ. Does alcohol increase the risk of preterm delivery? *Epidemiology.* 2000 Sep;11(5):512.

[155] Weile LK, Hegaard HK, Wu C, Tabor A, Wolf Trap H, Kesmodel US, Henriksen TB, Nohr E. Alcohol intake in early pregnancy and spontaneous preterm birth: A cohort study. doi:10.1111/ACER.1425.

[156] Patra J, Bakker R, Irving H, Jaddoe VW, Malini S, Rehm J (2011) Dose-response relationship between alcohol consumption before and during pregnancy and the risks of low birthweight, preterm birth and small for gestational age (SGA)-a systematic review and meta-analyses. *BJOG: an international journal of obstetrics and gynaecology* 118:1411- 1421.

[157] Pfinder M, Kunst AE, Feldmann R, van Eijsden M, Vrijkotte TG (2013) Preterm birth and small for gestational age in relation to alcohol consumption during pregnancy: stronger associations among vulnerable women? Results from two large Western-European studies. *BMC pregnancy and childbirth* 13:49.

[158] Albertsen K, Andersen AM, Olsen J, Gronbaek M (2004) Alcohol consumption during pregnancy and the risk of preterm delivery. *American journal of epidemiology* 159:155-161.

[159] Jaddoe VW, Bakker R, Hofman A, Mackenbach JP, Moll HA, Steegers EA, Witteman JC. Moderate alcohol consumption during pregnancy and the risk of low birthweight and preterm birth. The generation R study. *Ann Epidemiol.* 2007 Oct;17(10):834-40.

[160] Parazzini F, Chatenoud L, Surace M, Tozzi L, Salerio B, Bettoni G, Benzi G. Moderate alcohol drinking and risk of preterm birth. *Eur J Clin Nutr.* 2003 Oct;57(10):1345-9.

[161] Kuczkowski KM. Anesthetic implications of drug abuse in pregnancy. *J Clin Anesth.* 2003;15:382–394.

[162] Boer K, Smit BJ, van Huis AM, Hogerzeil HV. Substance use in pregnancy: do we care? *Acta Paediatr Suppl.* 1994 Nov;404:65-71.

[163] Slattery MM, Morrison JJ. Preterm Delivery. *Lancet* 2002;360: 1489-97.

[164] Vucinovic M, Roje D, Vucinovic Z, Capkun V, Bucat M, Banovic I. Maternal and neonatal effects of substance abuse during pregnancy: our ten-year experience. *Yonsei Med J.* 2008 Oct 31;49(5):705-13.

[165] Calhoun BC, Watson PT. The cost of maternal cocaine abuse: I. Perinatal cost. *Obstet Gynecol.* 1991 Nov;78(5 Pt 1):731-4.

[166] Sprauve ME, Lindsay MK, Herbert S, Graves W. Adverse perinatal outcome in parturients who use crack cocaine. *Obstet Gynecol.* 1997 May;89(5 Pt 1):674-8.

[167] Bada HS, Das A, Bauer CR, Shankaran S, Lester BM, Gard CC, Wright LL, Lagasse L, Higgins R. Low birth weight and preterm births: etiologic fraction attributable to prenatal drug exposure. *J Perinatol.* 2005 Oct;25(10):631-7.

[168] Cornelius MD, Taylor PM, Geva D, Day NL. Prenatal tobacco and marijuana use among adolescents: Effects on offspring gestational age, growth and morphology. *Pediatrics* 1995;95: 738–743.

[169] Fergusson DM, Horwood LJ, Northstone K; ALSPAC Study Team. Avon Longitudinal Study of Pregnancy and Childhood. Maternal use of cannabis and pregnancy outcome. *BJOG.* 2002 Jan;109(1):21-7.

In: Preterm Birth
Editors: A. Malik and A. Baarda
ISBN: 978-1-53618-298-9
© 2020 Nova Science Publishers, Inc.

Chapter 2

EPIDEMIOLOGICAL FACTORS FOR PRETERM BIRTH: PATERNAL AND FETAL FACTORS

Panos Antsaklis[1], MD, PhD,
Maria Papamichail[2,], MD,*
Marianna Theodora[3], MD, PhD
and George Daskalakis[4], MD, PhD

[1]Academic Fellow, 1st Department of Obstetrics and Gynecology, Department of Fetal Maternal Medicine, Alexandra Maternity Hospital, University of Athens, Athens, Greece
[2]Medical Doctor, Obstetrics and Gynecology trainee, Alexandra Maternity Hospital, University of Athens, Athens, Greece
[3]Lecturer, 1st Department of Obstetrics and Gynecology, Department of Fetal Maternal Medicine, Alexandra Maternity Hospital, University of Athens, Athens, Greece
[4]Associate Professor, 1st Department of Obstetrics and Gynecology, Department of Fetal Maternal Medicine, Alexandra Maternity Hospital, University of Athens, Athens, Greece

---

* Corresponding Author's E-mail: mapapam@hotmail.com.

ABSTRACT

Preterm birth is a global subject of interest, as WHO estimated that in 2014 more than 15 million neonates were born prematurely. Despite the enormous progress in neonatology, preterm birth remains a major obstetrical problem, being responsible for 65 - 75% of neonatal deaths and 75% of neonatal morbidity. Preterm birth has been characterized as an obstetrical syndrome, with multifactorial etiology and multiple pathophysiological mechanisms, in which the immune system and its responses playing a major role. In order to decrease the incidence of preterm birth and therefore to limit its consequences, it is important to try and understand this syndrome from an epidemiologic point of view, to detect the risk factors and when possible to avoid them. In the past years, maternal risk factors for preterm delivery were the most studied ones. However, some important risk factors concerning either the fetal or the paternal side, have been proved to be equally important. In this chapter, we will review the paternal risk factors including paternal anthropometric and genetic characteristics and life-style habits. In addition, fetal characteristics which may be responsible for increasing the risk of preterm birth will be discussed, including fetal sex, congenital anomalies and complications (i.e., severe I.U.G.R, fetal distress).

Keywords: epidemiology of preterm birth, paternal risk factors, fetal risk factors

1. INTRODUCTION

It is commonly accepted that preterm birth is a subject of global interest, as WHO estimated that in 2014 more than 15 million neonates were born prematurely. Despite the major progress in neonatology, preterm birth is responsible for 65 - 75% of neonatal deaths and 75% of neonatal morbidity [1]. In the past years, many trials and surveys studied the maternal factors that increase the risk for preterm birth, in order to identify high risk women for preterm birth and when possible to modify these risk factors in order to decrease their possibility for preterm delivery. On the other hand, trials studying the risk factors concerning either the father or the fetus are very limited. Additionally, their results might be biased, as many of their data are taken retrospectively and only through questionnaires that were answered by the mothers.

According to many studies, preterm birth has been characterized as an obstetrical syndrome with multifactorial etiology and multiple pathophysiological mechanisms, in which the immune system and its responses playing a major role. Paternal factors might be equally important to the interaction of these mechanisms, as they could influence birth outcomes through a number of pathways acting indirectly through maternal factors. For example, paternal education and paternal support-involvement during the period of pregnancy it is well proved that they have a major impact on mother's health behaviors, such as smoking during pregnancy, adequate antenatal care and timely antenatal visits and finally stress limitation, factors that are responsible for increased preterm birth rates. Additionally, paternal life style and support play a key role to the quality of the maternal environment and therefore indirectly affect the fetal environment. Finally, paternal DNA contributes to the 50% of the newborn's genome and there is evidence suggesting that paternal genetic components are significant for the embryo quality and fetal development [2-4].

In this chapter, an overview of the most important paternal risk factors for preterm birth, such as paternal age, birth-weight, education and occupation will be presented. Additionally, we will present the fetal risk factors that may increase the incidence of preterm birth, specifically fetal sex, congenital anomalies and sex disorders. Finally, the possible explanations for the significance of these factors will be discussed, aiming to the better understanding of the pathophysiology of preterm birth.

2. PATERNAL RISK FACTORS

2.1. Paternal Anthropometric Characteristics (Age, Height, Weight, Birth-Weight)

In the current literature, there are contradictory results concerning the correlation between paternal age and preterm birth. Some surveys failed to associate paternal weight with higher preterm birth rates [5-10], while other studies found that advanced paternal age is a risk factor for preterm birth.

More specifically, Astofli et al. [11] claimed that paternal age ranging from 45 to 49 years old is associated with a 1.91 and 1.72 times higher risk for having babies born very preterm and moderately preterm respectively, when compared to fathers aged 25 - 29 years old. These numbers were in line with Zhu's et al. [12] trial, which showed that fathers older than 50 years had 2.1 times higher risk for having preterm neonates.

The authors also suggested that the more advanced the paternal age, the greater the risk for preterm birth. Furthermore, in a recent study, Goisis et al. [13] found a U-shaped association between paternal age and preterm birth, with fathers belonging in the 30 - 34 age group, having the lowest preterm birth rates.

Finally, in a trial run in the USA and studied 9 million births, it was showed that white women whose partner was much younger than them, had the highest risks for preterm birth. Interestingly, this observation was not valid for black women [14].

According to Shah [15] paternal age, weight and height are not associated with a higher possibility for preterm birth. Interestingly, according to Klebanoff et al. [16], neonates whose father's birth weight was more than 4kg, were more likely to be born prematurely. However, this finding might be biased by several maternal factors that were not included in the risk model of this study.

2.2. Paternal Educational Level

Paternal education is one of the strongest contributors for preterm birth, as many authors claimed that paternal education is a better indicator for the family's socioeconomic status than maternal educational level. In Parker and Schoendorf's study [17], it was clearly noticed that the higher the educational level, the lower the risk for preterm birth. In numbers, when the father had not graduated from high school, the odds ratio for preterm birth was 1.53, while when the father was a high school graduator the risk was 1.28 times higher, compared to fathers who were college graduators.

Shapiro et al. [37] consorted with the study above, as in their trial found that fathers without a high school degree, showed an increased risk for preterm birth with an odds ratio of 1.22. This risk climbed to 1.37 when the mother also had a low educational level. Finally, Meng and Groth counted a 34.6% higher risk for preterm birth among fathers without high school degree and a 22.6% higher risk among high school graduators fathers, compared with fathers having a higher than a high school degree [10].

Concerning the mechanisms responsible for this finding and considering the biopsychosocial contributors of preterm birth, the pregnant wives of highly educated fathers are more likely to enjoy increased paternal support and adequate antenatal care, factors that can lead to a decline of the preterm birth rates.

2.3. Paternal Occupation

Several studies failed to prove any correlation between parental occupation and preterm birth [18-21]. Nevertheless, Savitz et al. [22] studied the paternal x-ray exposure and they found a 1.5 times higher risk for preterm birth among neonates whose father was exposed to x-rays, in comparison to non-exposed fathers.

Additionally, prolonged lead exposure elevates the possibility for preterm birth by about 5 times [23]. As mentioned in our previous chapter, maternal environmental exposure on lead and other air pollutants, also increase the risk for preterm birth.

Therefore, it is reasonable to think that either paternal behavior and therefor exposure can lead consequently to increased maternal exposure as well and *vice versa*, or there could be a gene modification in the germ cell line caused by this parental exposure, leading to abnormalities on fertility, conception and placentation [15].

2.4. Paternal Involvement

Concerning paternal involvement, Alio et al. [14] found that in teen pregnancies, parental presence and support to the future mother is a protective factor for preterm birth. In numbers, babies whose father was in any way absent during the pregnancy period, had 1.49 times higher risk to be born very prematurely. Possible explanations for these findings, is the fact that women who experience their pregnancy having good support by their partner-father are more likely to attend their antenatal appointments regularly and also to omit harmful behaviors during pregnancy, such as smoking and alcohol consumption. Additionally, when a woman enjoys support and care from her partner, she is relieved from stress and the pregnancy complications that may be caused by it.

2.5. Partner Alteration

According to Vatten et al. [25] women who changed partners between two pregnancies, have to be considered as a high-risk group for preterm birth, concerning the second pregnancy. This remark hides significant importance, as divorces and new marriages are very common the last decades. Interestingly, despite the fact that women with higher educational level are less likely to deliver preterm, in this trial, women with high educational level and different partners, had higher risk for preterm birth, compared to low-educated women who also changed their partner. However, it is debatable whether partner changing contributes to increased preterm birth rate as an independent risk factor or if it reflects other social characteristics, that also increase preterm birth risk, such as advanced maternal age, smoking and long interpregnancy intervals. This observation has been studied and tried to be explained through paternal genes and antigens interaction, without conclusive results [26-27].

Concerning women who already had one preterm birth and then had a second pregnancy with a different partner, their risk for preterm birth was not decreased, concluding that paternal impact on preterm birth risk is not significant [26]. In contrast, Li et al. [27] suggested that partner alteration leads to a small reduction of the risk for preterm birth for women who had a previous preterm birth before the 34th gestational week. The risk remained the same for women with previous delivery between the 34th-36th gestational week, while for women delivering after the 36th weeks, the risk was elevated. This finding shows that the impact of partner changing depends on the outcome of the previous pregnancy and it might be associated with the paternal human leukocyte antigen (HLA). In addition, Ness et al. [32] suggested that male reproductive proteins (MRPs) that are found in the sperm, could change the vaginal flora, making women vulnerable to infections and therefore to preterm birth.

3. FETAL RISK FACTORS

3.1. Fetal Sex

It is well known that male fetuses present higher rates of mortality and morbidity compared to female fetuses [28-29]. Additionally, many studies have related fetal sex with preterm birth, a finding that could explain the previous observation [28]. According to Brettel et al. [29] male infants are 1.31 times more likely to be born prematurely after spontaneous preterm birth, than female infants.

However, the risk for iatrogenic preterm birth was not statistically significantly different between the two genders, finding which is in line with Zeitlin's et al. [30] trial. Ingemarsson recorded and sub-grouped births according to the gestational duration and fetal sex and he noticed that more male neonates were born before the 37th week of gestation than female [31]. The association between preterm birth and male sex is also valid in twin pregnancies. Tan et al. [33] found that the highest rates of preterm birth among twin pregnancies were presented in pregnancies with two male fetuses, compared to female-female or male-female pairs. The risk for preterm birth was 4.9%, 12.4% and 40.2% for preterm birth before the 28th, 32nd and 36th week respectively.

The fact that male infants are more likely to be born prematurely could be explained by the following: 1) male infants tend to weight more, leading to bigger uterus expansion [34] and 2) women carrying male infants, have higher levels of interleukin-1, a pro-inflammatory cytokine, which could be related to premature labor.

3.2. Congenital Anomalies and Pregnancy Complications

DeFranco et al. [35] studied the impact of congenital anomalies and fetal sex disorders on preterm birth. They founded that fetuses with congenital anomalies and sex disorders presented 5.4 and 5.1 times higher risk for preterm birth respectively. The scientist did not mention the type or the severity of the anomalies. Jiang et al. [36] run a study in Taiwan and they studied maternal and fetal characteristics among 2,652 births. They sub-grouped neonates in to two teams; the first group included babies who were born at term and the second group included babies who were born prematurely. The authors found that fetal growth restriction rate was greater in the preterm birth group, while oligohydramnios, hydramnios or fetal distress were not statistically different between the two teams.

CONCLUSION

In conclusion, there is no doubt that preterm birth is responsible for the largest percentage of neonatal morbidity and mortality. Concerning the emanation of preterm birth, the scientific community is doubting between the interaction of several pathways and the independent effect of one major pathway. In order to make reality the prevention and prediction of preterm birth, we have to detect firstly the risk factors and the parental characteristics increasing preterm birth incidence. In this chapter we provided an overview of most paternal and fetal factors that could play a role on the preterm birth occurrence and that often may lack the appropriate attention. Finally, it is important to mention that further research is necessary in order to detect other possible, still unknown risk factors for preterm birth. Ideally, a complete medical and socio-economical profile, including detailed demographic characteristics of each pregnant women should be carried out during each pregnancy. By this way women who are at high risk for preterm birth could be identified and the aim would be not only to detect these women in order to offer them a more strict antenatal care, but also when possible to modify any of these risk factors in order to decrease the preterm birth incidence.

REFERENCES

[1] Chawanpaiboon, S. et al. Global, regional, and national estimates of levels of preterm birth in 2014: a systematic review and modelling analysis. *Lancet Glob. Health,* 2019; 7: e37 - 46.

[2] Constantinof, A., Moisiadis, V. G., and Matthews, S. G. (2016). Programming of stress pathways: A transgenerational perspective. *The Journal of Steroid Biochemistry and Molecular Biology,* 160, 175 - 180.

[3] Yang, Q., Zhao, F., Dai, S., Zhang, N., Zhao, W., Bai, R., and Sun, Y. (2015). Sperm telomere length is positively associated with the quality of early embryonic development. *Human Reproduction,* 30(8), 1876 - 1881.

[4] Yuan, S., Schuster, A., Tang, C., Yu, T., Ortogero, N., Bao, J., ... Yan, W. (2016). Sperm-borne miRNAs and endo-siRNAs are important for fertilization and preimplantation embryonic development. *Development,* 143(4), 635 - 647.

[5] Chen, X. K., Wen, S. W., Krewski, D. et al. Paternal age and adverse birth outcomes: teenager or 40+, who is at risk? *Hum. Reprod.,* 2008; 23:1290 - 6.

[6] Abel, E. L., Kruger, M., Burd, L. Effects of maternal and paternal age on Caucasian and Native American preterm births and birth weights. *Am. J. Perinatol.,* 2002; 19:049 - 54.

[7] Basso, O., Wilcox, A. J. Paternal age and delivery before 32 weeks. *Epidemiology,* 2006; 17:475 - 8.

[8] Nahum, G. G., Stanislaw, H. Relationship of paternal factors to birth weight. *J. Reprod. Med.,* 2003; 48:963 - 8.

[9] Tough, S. C., Faber, A. J., Svenson, L. W. et al. Is paternal age associated with an increased risk of low birthweight, preterm delivery, and multiple birth? *Can. J. Public Health,* 2003; 94:88 - 92.

[10] Meng, Y., Groth, S. W. Fathers Count: The Impact of Paternal Risk Factors on Birth Outcomes. *Matern. Child Health J.,* 2018; Mar.; 22(3):401 - 408. doi: 10.1007/s10995-017-2407-8.

[11] Astolfi, P., De Pasquale, A., Zonta, L. A. Paternal age and preterm birth in Italy, 1990 to 1998. *Epidemiology,* 2006; 17:218 - 21.

[12] Zhu, J. L., Madsen, K. M., Vestergaard, M. et al. Paternal age and preterm birth. *Epidemiology,* 2005; 16:259 - 62.

[13] Goisis, A., Remes, H., Barclay, K. et al. *J. Epidemiol. Community Health,* Epub ahead of print: [please include Day Month Year]. doi:10.1136/jech-2017- 210170.

[14] Kinzler, W. L., Ananth, C. V., Smulian, J. C. et al. Parental age difference and adverse perinatal outcomes in the United States. *Paediatr. Perinat. Epidemiology,* 2002; 16:297 - 304.

[15] Shah, P. S. Paternal factors and low birthweight, preterm, and small for gestational age births: a systematic review. *Am. J. Obstet. Gynecol.,* 2010 Feb.; 202(2):103 - 23.

[16] Klebanoff, M. A., Mednick, B. R., Schulsinger, C., Secher, N. J., Shiono, P. H. Father's effect on infant birth weight. *Am. J. Obstet. Gynecol.,* 1998; 178:1022 - 6.

[17] Parker, J. D., Schoendorf, K. C. Influence of paternal characteristics on the risk of low birth weight. *Am. J. Epidemiol.,* 1992; 136:399 - 407.

[18] Lawson, C. C., Schnorr, T. M., Whelan, E. A. et al. Paternal occupational exposure to 2,3,7,8-tetrachlorodibenzo- p-dioxin and birth outcomes of offspring: birth weight, preterm delivery, and birth defects. *Environ. Health Perspect,* 2004; 112:1403 - 8.

[19] Lin, S., Hwang, S. A., Marshall, E. G., Marion, D. Does paternal occupational lead exposure increase the risks of low birth weight or prematurity? *Am. J. Epidemiol.,* 1998; 148:173 - 81.

[20] Mjoen, G., Saetre, D. O., Lie, R. T. et al. Paternal occupational exposure to radiofrequency electromagnetic fields and risk of adverse pregnancy outcome. *Eur. J. Epidemiol.,* 2006; 21: 529 - 35.

[21] Sanjose, S., Roman, E., Beral, V. Low birthweight and preterm delivery, Scotland, 1981 - 84: effect of parents' occupation. *Lancet,* 1991; 338:428 - 31.

[22] Savitz, D. A., Whelan, E. A., Kleckner, R. C. Effect of parents' occupational exposures on risk of stillbirth, preterm delivery, and small-for-gestational-age infants. *Am. J. Epidemiol.,* 1989; 129: 1201 - 18.

[23] Min, Y. I., Correa-Villasenor, A., Stewart, P. A. Parental occupational lead exposure and low birth weight. *Am. J. Ind. Med.,* 1996; 30:569 - 78.

[24] Alio, A. P., Mbah, A. K., Grunsten, R. A., Salihu, H. M. Teenage pregnancy and the influence of paternal involvement on fetal outcomes. *J. Pediatr. Adolesc. Gynecol.,* 2011; Dec.; 24(6):404 - 9.

[25] Vatten, L. J., Skjaerven, R. Effects on pregnancy outcome of changing partner between first two births: prospective population study. *BMJ,* 2003; Nov. 15; 327(7424):1138.

[26] Basso, O., Olsen, J., Christensen, K. Study of environmental, social, and paternal factors in preterm delivery using sibs and half sibs. A population-based study in Denmark. *J. Epidemiol. Community Health,* 1999; Jan.; 53(1):20 - 3.

[27] Li, D. K. Changing paternity and the risk of preterm delivery in the subsequent pregnancy. *Epidemiology,* 1999; 10: 148 - 52.

[28] Zeitlin, J., Saurel-Cubizolles, M. J., De Mouzon, J., Rivera, L., Ancel, P. Y., Blondel, B., Kaminski, M. Fetal sex and preterm birth: are males at greater risk? *Hum. Reprod.,* 2002; Oct.; 17(10):2762 - 8.

[29] Brettell, R., Yeh, P. S., Impey, L. W. Examination of the association between male gender and preterm delivery. *Eur. J. Obstet. Gynecol. Reprod. Biol.,* 2008; Dec.; 141(2):123 - 6.

[30] Zeitlin, J., Ancel, P. Y., Larroque, B., Kaminski, M.; EPIPAGE Study. Fetal sex and indicated very preterm birth: results of the EPIPAGE study. *Am. J. Obstet. Gynecol.,* 2004; May;190(5): 1322 - 5.

[31] Ingemarsson, I. Gender aspects of preterm birth. *BJOG,* 2003; Apr.; 110 Suppl. 20:34 - 8.

[32] Ness, R. B., Grainger, D. A. Male reproductive proteins and reproductive outcomes. *Am. J. Obstet. Gynecol.,* 2008; Jun.; 198(6):620.e1 - 4.

[33] Tan, H., Wen, S. W., Walker, M., Fung, K. F., Demissie, K., Rhoads, G. G. The association between fetal sex and preterm birth in twin pregnancies. *Obstet. Gynecol.,* 2004; Feb.; 103(2):327 - 32.

[34] McGregor, J. A., Leff, M., Orleans, M., Baron, A. Fetal gender differences in preterm birth: findings in a North American cohort. *Am. J. Perinatol.,* 1992; Jan.; 9(1):43 - 8.

[35] DeFranco, E., Hall, E., Muglia, L. Racial Disparity in Previable Birth. *Am. J. Obstet. Gynecol.,* 2016; Mar.; 214 (3), 394.e1 - 7.

[36] Min Jiang, Miskatul Mustafa Mishu, Dan Lu, Xianghua Yin. A Case Control Study of Risk Factors and Neonatal Outcomes of Preterm Birth. *Taiwan J. Obstet. Gynecol.,* 2018, Dec; 57 (6), 814 - 818.

[37] Shapiro, G. D., Bushnik, T., Sheppard, A. J. et al. *J. Epidemiol. Community Health,* 2017; 71:67 - 72.

Chapter 3

THE LINK BETWEEN DHA AND BONE TURNOVER IN THE PRETERM NEONATE

Javier Diaz-Castro[1,2,*], Jorge Moreno-Fernandez[1,2] and Julio J. Ochoa[1,2]

[1]Departament of Physiology, Faculty of Pharmacy, University of Granada, Granada, Spain
[2]Institute of Nutrition and Food Technology "José Mataix Verdú," Biomedical Research Center, Health Sciences Technological Park, University of Granada, Granada, Spain

ABSTRACT

According to the World Health Organization, 10% of the world's births occur before the 37th week of gestation. A significant increase in the survival rate of preterm infants has been reported in recent decades. In parallel, this has increased emerging conditions, such as osteopenia of prematurity, which can occur in up to 30% of infants born before the 28th week of gestation. The prevalence depends on gestational age, weight and type of diet. It occurs in 55% of premature babies weighing less than

---

[*] Corresponding Author's E-mail: javierdc@ugr.es.

1,000 g and in 23% of infants weighing less than 1,500 g at birth. Osteopenia of the newborn is characterized by the reduction of bone mineral content, and is caused both by severe nutritional deficiencies and by biomechanical factors. It occurs between the tenth and sixteenth weeks of life, but may not be detected until there is severe demineralization (between 20 and 40% loss of bone mineral). Despite being a common disease, there are important controversies in the literature regarding the methods of detection of infants at risk, as well as their interpretation. The prevention of osteopenia of the preterm newborn and its timely treatment should be the primary objective of health. In this sense, ω-3 polyunsaturated fatty acids (ω-3 PUFA) are a group of fatty acids (FA) that are essential components of the human diet because they cannot be synthesized. Three important omega-3 fatty acids are alpha-linolenic acid (ALA), eicosapentaenoic acid (EPA), and docosahexaenoic acid (DHA). Sources of EPA and DHA are fatty fish such as salmon, fish oil supplements, or the conversion of ingested alpha-linolenic acid to DHA or EPA, though evidence reports that the conversion rate is low, especially in the neonate. ω-3 PUFA play an important role in bone metabolism and may represent a useful non-pharmacological way of ameliorating bone loss and risk of osteoporosis. ω-3 is precursor for several potent regulatory eicosanoids involved in bone metabolism including PG and leukotrienes. Thereby, ω-3 PUFA can inhibit the production of these inflammatory cytokines such as IL-1, IL-6 and TNF-α, which provide an important stimulus for osteoclastic bone resorption, and suppression of the production of these cytokines by n-3 PUFA may inhibit bone resorption and prevent bone loss.

Keywords: preterm neonates, bone turnover, DHA

INTRODUCTION

There are several determinants that can affect pregnancy such as socioeconomic status, family structure, housing quality, access to healthy food, access to health and primary care services, health technology, social cohesion, perception of discrimination/inequality, access to employment, employment status, policies that support health promotion, safe school environments and admission to higher education (Maness and Buhi 2016). Prematurity is one of the results of these health determinants, which also becomes an important determinant of neonatal mortality and morbidity, with long-term consequences (Wang et al. 2004). Children born prematurely not only have higher mortality and morbidity in the neonatal period, but later in life, resulting in enormous costs (Petrou, 2005), hence it is conceived as a high priority for public health in some countries.

According to the World Health Organization, 10% of the world's births occur before the 37th week of gestation (WHO 2012). A significant increase in the survival rate of preterm infants has been reported in recent decades. In parallel, this has increased emerging conditions, such as osteopenia of prematurity, which can occur in up to 30% of infants born before the 28th week of gestation. The prevalence depends on gestational age, weight and type of diet. It occurs in 55% of premature babies weighing less than 1,000 g and in 23% of infants weighing less than 1,500 g at birth. Osteopenia of the newborn is characterized by the reduction of bone mineral content, and is caused both by severe nutritional deficiencies and by biomechanical factors. It occurs between the tenth and sixteenth weeks of life, but may not be detected until there is severe demineralization (between 20 and 40% loss of bone mineral) (Bozzetti and Tagliabue 2009). Despite being a common disease, there are important controversies in the literature regarding the methods of detection of infants at risk, as well as their interpretation (Harrison and Gibson 2013).

PRETERM NEONATE: EPIDEMIOLOGY AND CLINICAL OUTCOMES

Preterm birth is the biggest clinical challenge currently facing perinatal medicine. The biggest amount of neonatal deaths occur in premature newborns, and prematurity is a high risk factor for deficiency and disability, with many family and social repercussions. There is an increase in the prematurity rate in developed countries. This is a challenge which changes the healthcare practice to these neonates, allowing advances from obstetric and neonatal care, which improves neonatal survival of preterm neonates. From the statistical point of view the limitation must be taken into account of the traditional classification in abortion, fetal death and early neonatal death, and of the different national laws, that establish mandatory limits of record, with descending gestational age, according to the survivals achieved (Tucker and McGuire 2004).

The delivery should take place in a hospital environment, preferably scheduled with the presence of a neonatologist and an expert nurse. All the necessary material for resuscitation and transfer in a stable thermal environment, provided with assistance support to provide mechanical ventilation, should be avilable, maintaining perfusion and continuous monitoring of oxygen saturation and heart rate by pulse oximetry. There are studies that show that the use of continuous positive airway pressure for the initial stabilization of premature newborns has been accompanied by a decrease in surfactant use and the number of days with oxygen supply (Huddleston, Sanchez-Ramos, and Huddleston 2003).

Most premature babies are born after the presentation of a spontaneous preterm birth or born after premature amniorrexis (>50%). The presence of clinical or subclinical infection is suspected (positive cultures in the fetal annexes in 60% versus 20% of the term; maternal vaginosis, elevated inflammatory markers in amniotic fluid), although antibacterial treatment is not effective in childbirth spontaneous premature. On the contrary, its use in premature amniorrexis manages to prolong pregnancy, decrease the rate of choriomnionitis and improve neonatal outcomes (Jain and Cheng 2006).

Other associated factors with prematurity are: the existence of previous preterm births, the unfavorable socioeconomic situation of the mother and maternal smoking. Measures that improve antenatal, medical, dietary and social care are effective in correcting inequality and controlling the prematurity rate.

Multiple spontaneous or induced pregnancy increase prematurity rates and accounts for approximately a quarter of the preterm. The incidence of twins and triplets multiplied in the first years of development of assisted reproduction techniques. More than 50% of twins and almost all triplets and multiples are preterm infants. Maternal and fetal complications are the cause of 15 and 25% of preterm. The highest percentage is represented by maternal hypertension and intrauterine malnutrition, followed by polyhydramnios. Prematurity is obstetrically induced in certain fetal pathologies such as diabetic fetopathy, fetal hydrops etc. Premature newborns are in danger of developing multiple nutritional deficiencies (Rustico, Calabria, and Garber 2014).

BONE TURNOVER

Bones is a metabolically active tissue that undergoes continuous remodelling to cope with the body's Ca requirements and to repair microscopic damage in a dynamic process where osteoblasts are responsible for bone formation and osteoclasts for its resorption. These processes rely on the activity of osteoclasts (resorption), osteoblasts (formation) and osteocytes (maintenance). Under normal conditions, bone resorption and formation are tightly coupled to each other, so that the amount of bone removed is always equal to the amount of newly formed bone. The entire skeleton is replaced every 10 years in adults, and around 10% of the skeleton is involved in bone remodelling at any one time. This balance or turnover is achieved and regulated through the action of several hormones (PTH, PTH-related peptide [PTHrP], vitamin D, osteocalcin, alkaline phosphatase…) and local mediators (cytokines, growth factors…). In contrast, growth, ageing, metabolic bone diseases, states of increased or decreased mobility, therapeutic interventions, nutritional deficiencies and many other conditions are characterized by imbalances in bone turnover. The results of such uncoupling in bone turnover are often changes in bone structure, strength, mineralization and mass.

Osteoblasts are specialized mesenchymal cells that have also a role in the regulation of bone resorption through receptor activator of nuclear factor-kB (RANK) ligand (RANKL), that links to its receptor, RANK, on the surface of pre-osteoclast cells, inducing their differentiation and fusion. On the other hand, osteoblasts secrete a soluble decoy receptor (osteoprotegerin, OPG) that blocks RANK/RANKL interaction by binding to RANKL and, thus, prevents osteoclast differentiation and activation.

Therefore, the balance between RANKL and OPG determines the formation and activity of osteoclasts (Caetano-Lopes, Canhao, and Fonseca 2007).

Osteoclasts are the cells that degrade (resorb) bone during normal bone remodeling and in pathologic states in which bone resorption is increased. Osteoclasts form microscopic trenches on the surfaces of bone trabeculae in the spongy bone by secreting hydrochloric acid and proteases, such as cathepsin K, into an extracellular lyzosomal compartment beneath a ruffled part of their basal cell membrane to dissolve the mineral and matrix components of bone simultaneously. Precursors of osteoblasts, the cells that form bone, are recruited to these trenches from the adjacent bone marrow stromal cell population and differentiate into osteoblasts, which lay down new matrix and mineralize it (Boyce, Yao, and Xing 2009). Bone remodeling can be increased in response to many influences, including mechanical strain, cytokines, hormones, growth and dietary factors.

Bone remodeling occurs at discrete sites within the skeleton and is triggered in response to mechanical strain. Osteocytes are specialized "mechano-sensing" cells that reside within bone matrix. They detect mechanical strain and initiate signaling pathways, leading to both osteoclastogenesis and osteoblastogenesis (Poulsen, Moughan, and Kruger 2007). Lipid mediators have a critical role in the signaling pathway. Within seconds after mechanical loading of bone, the lipid mediator prostaglandin E2 (PGE_2) is released by osteocytes and mature osteoblasts (Bonewald 2006). Phospholipase-mediated membrane release fatty acids, notably arachidonic acid (AA, 20:4n- 6), the substrate for PGE_2 synthesis, and expression of the inducible form of cyclooxygenase (COX), COX-2, which oxidizes AA to PGE_2, are upregulated as an early response to strain (Smith and Clark 2005). PGE_2 promotes osteoclastogenesis by stimulating expression of both RANK-L and RANK and inhibiting expression of OPG. PGE_2 also activates the Wnt signaling pathway and promotes core binding factor α-1 (cbfa-1) and insulin-like growth factor 1 (IGF-1) expression, thereby stimulating osteoblastogenesis (Yoshida et al. 2002). PGE_2 are potent modulators of bone remodeling, affecting bone resorption, by stimulating osteoclastogenesis through RANKL. Both processes, formation and resorption, are related to PGE_2, and its effects on bone may be dose-dependent. At low levels, PGE_2 stimulates bone formation by osteoblasts, whereas high levels suppress osteoblast, promotes differentiation and bone resorption by osteoclasts, via RANKL (Griel et al. 2007).

BONE TURNOVER DURING PREGNANCY, LACTATION AND NEWBORN DEVELOPMENT

The process of bone remodeling begins in early life, in the uterus, and continues throughout the life of the individual. During childhood and adolescence, the formation process exceeds resorption, resulting in the acquisition of bone, both in length and in diameter; they change shape, increasing their mass and density, reaching a maximum that is reached between 30 and 40 years of age (Indumati, Patil, and Jailkhani 2007). Gestation and lactation are two stages in the life of women in which physiological adaptations occur, which include changes in bone metabolism, as compensatory mechanisms to ensure adequate mineral development of the fetus and the necessary protection to the skeleton maternal (Glerean and Plantalech 2000).

The kidneys, intestine and skeleton (through bone resorption) are not the main sources that supply minerals in the fetus, as in the adult. Instead, the placenta responds to the need of the fetus by active transport of calcium, phosphorus, and magnesium from the maternal circulation. This occurs especially during the third trimester of pregnancy, in order to ossify the collagen matrix of the fetal skeleton before birth (Kovacs 2014). During pregnancy, the increase in calcium demands is maintained by the improvement of intestinal absorption, mediated by vitamin D (Yoon et al. 2000). The availability of minerals also influences the function and activity of osteoblasts and osteoclasts (Kovacs 2014).

Bone and mineral metabolism in the fetus are directly linked with PTH and parathyroid hormone-related protein (PTHrP), since both are required for placental calcium transfer; while vitamin D/calcitriol, FGF23

(Fibroblast growth factor 23), calcitonin, and sex steroids, are not as necessary as PTH is (Kovacs 2014). In fact, PTH levels are slightly decreased in the first trimester and normal in the other two, which may represent a modest suppression of the parathyroid gland at the beginning of pregnancy. But PTHrP levels seem to contribute to the functional state of maternal hyperparathyroidism, which maintains the necessary maternal-fetal calcium gradient, in addition to regulating the formation of endochondral bone in humans (Glerean and Plantalech 2000).

In the early stages of pregnancy, the concentration of osteocalcin is decreased and then increases from the third trimester of pregnancy and remains elevated during the lactation stage, which reflects the high bone turnover that occurs in the mother, which would contribute to the calcium intake necessary for skeletal maturation of the fetus and newborn (Glerean and Plantalech 2000). Yoon et al. (2000), (Yoon et al. 2000) found osteocalcin levels significantly reduced at 16 weeks gestation and then elevated at 6 weeks postpartum; as well as a marker of bone resorption (deoxypyridine) increased from the second trimester.

During the last trimester of pregnancy, there is an exponential increase in bone formation, in which 80% of the fetal bone is produced, while the total calcium in the bone increases from approximately 5 g at week 24 to 30 g at the end. The peak of the bone accumulation rate occurs around 32 weeks of gestation. To meet this high demand for calcium and phosphorus in this period of rapid bone formation during the last trimester, there is a placental active transport of calcium and phosphorus from the mother to the fetus (Kovacs 2011). This decrease in total calcium in the mother is considered between 5 and 6% of the pre-pregnancy level reaching a valley in the middle of the third trimester and then increases slightly (Glerean and Plantalech 2000).

Intestinal calcium absorption doubles during pregnancy, particularly in the last trimester. Urinary calcium excretion is also increased proportionally to the glomerular filtration rate. The increase in the synthesis of active metabolites of vitamin D, elevated prolactin secretion and intestinal hypertrophy produced seem to contribute to this state of intestinal hyperabsorption and hypercalciuria (Glerean and Plantalech

2000). Gertner et al. (1986), (Gertner et al. 1986) evaluated the response of calcemia to oral calcium intake in women in their third trimester of pregnancy.

After pregnancy, breastfeeding continues to demand more calcium to concentrate in breast milk. To compensate for the greater increase in calcium by the production of breast milk, maternal adaptations include both bone resorption and renal reabsorption of calcium, a mechanism that is evident until the sixth month post-lactation. Several studies find that nursing women have a tendency to greater resorption compared to non-lactating women (Yoon et al. 2000).

These physiological compensatory mechanisms allow, in most cases, to cope with the necessary requirements for the formation and mineralization of the fetal skeleton and the nutrition of the newborn, overcoming this period without major difficulties. However, some women experience bone demineralization that can be complicated by fractures and a small group undergoes regional demineralization. Osteoporosis associated with pregnancy or breastfeeding is a rare complication that can cause clinical problems in susceptible women. Repeated pregnancies may increase the risk of osteoporosis in these women with low bone density, especially associated with prolonged breastfeeding (Yoon et al. 2000).

According to the Utah paradigm (Frost 1997), the bone is formed in two stages: a first stage of skeletal system embryogenesis and a second stage of bone formation that begins in the second half of the second trimester. Diametral growth in long bones occurs through models in which osteoclasts remove the bone from the endostium and osteoblasts form bone along the periosteum.

During childhood, especially in the first four years of life, it is the moment in which the phenomena of bone turnover reach their maximum intensity. This is manifested by high levels of osteocalcin and serum propeptide. Umbilical cord blood usually contains low levels of PTH and calcitriol, normal or low levels of FGF23, and high levels of PTHrP and calcitonin. After birth, calcium in the blood drops by 20-30%, followed by an increase during the next 24 hours, where adult levels are reached; the increase in PTH precedes an increase in calcitrol (Kovacs 2011).

Premature infants will not receive the important maternal contribution of calcium and phosphorus in recent months, so they have a lower bone mineral content than full-term newborns. On the other hand, due to prematurity, they can present a non-glandular response by the parathyroid. Likewise, the contributions of exogenous calcium and phosphorus are not always sufficient because it receives small volumes of breast milk and the cutaneous synthesis of Vitamin D is also diminished by the low solar radiation that these newborns receive. It is currently well established that more than calcium, phosphate levels are critical for the proper deposition of minerals in the bone matrix, therefore, in most premature infants it is necessary to supplement breast milk or use formulas for prematurity, to ensure sufficient mineral intake to complete adequate bone mineralization (Kovacs 2014).

Intestinal calcium absorption in the newborn (especially in premature babies) is largely a passive process and facilitated by the high lactose content of breast milk. This is why premature babies do not respond to calcitriol, but initially depend on passive mineral absorption. As the neonate matures, intestinal calcium absorption (dependent on calcitriol) becomes the dominant mechanism (Kovacs 2014). Metabolic bone disease (MBD) is a relatively frequent problem, observed in the evolution of premature newborns. Among the problems related to the feeding of premature infants, bone mineralization alterations have been noted for their high incidence. The generalized finding that the bones of premature babies are shorter and lighter, and contain less calcium per unit length than those of the fetus and the newborn at term of equivalent post-conceptional ages, motivated interest in the study of the peculiarities of mineral metabolism in this group of neonates (Rustico, Calabria, and Garber 2014).

MBD of prematurity is an increasingly frequent process or group of diagnostic processes in infants of lower gestational age and neonatal weight, whose common and defining characteristic is the presence of an alteration of bone mineralization, which can go from the simple decrease of the mineral content (osteopenia), to the severe affectation of the same with rickety changes in the distal extremities of the long bones and bone fractures. In its genesis different factors are involved, some not well known, although at present, it is considered that the common origin of these disorders lies in the lower incorporation of calcium into the bone achieved with enteral feeding, compared to that provided by the transplacental mineral flow during the third trimester of pregnancy (Chan, Mileur, and Hansen 1988). As MBD advances, biochemical changes intensify. These changes commonly include hypophosphatemia, hyperphosphatasia, and secondary hyperparathyroidism, which may be accompanied by rachitic changes and/or fractures. Inadequate bone mineralization during this period may compromise pulmonary status and contribute to poor growth (Rustico, Calabria, and Garber 2014).

In summary, the fetal and neonatal skeleton requires adequate mineral content in order to develop and mineralize normally. Both PTH and PTHrP are essential for maintaining high serum levels of calcium and phosphorus in the uterus, for optimal bone mineralization. Similarly, the development of endochondral bone during fetal development requires PTH and PTHrP, but not calcitriol, calcitonin or sex steroids. It is in the neonatal period when intestinal calcium absorption and, therefore, skeletal development and mineralization become dependent on vitamin D/calcitriol. During breastfeeding, most studies have shown an increase in bone remodeling. This may happen in part due to a decrease in plasma estradiol and an increase in plasma prolactin and PTHrP during breastfeeding (Kovacs 2014).

ROLE OF ω-3 FATTY ACIDS IN PRETERM NEONATE BONE TURNOVER

In the study developed by Kajarabille et al. (2018), (Kajarabille et al. 2018) a group of mothers and their healthy term neonates were enrolled in a registered, double blind, controlled study, from the sixth month gestation to the fourth month of neonate's life. 110 pregnant women were recruited. Women were randomly assigned to one of the following intervention groups following an unpredictable sequence computer-generated: DHA group: consumption of 400 mL/day of fish oil enriched dairy drink; Control group: consumption of 400 mL/day of the control dairy drink. This study revealed that in pregnant mothers, DHA supplementation increased osteocalcin (OC) and osteopontin (OPN) levels and decreased IL-6 and TNF-α levels at delivery, increasing PTH levels during lactation. In neonates, DHA supplementation increased ACTH, insulin and leptin, decreasing RANKL and IL-6 in umbilical vein; increased OPG and leptin and diminished TNF-α in umbilical artery; increased OC levels, lowered PTH and TNF-α at birth. The role of omega-3 LC PUFA in bone health is a relatively new subject of study and virtually non-existent in pregnant women and neonates. The study of Karabille et al. (2018) (Kajarabille et al. 2018) was the first study evaluating the effect of omega-3 LC PUFA on bone metabolism in both, the mother and the neonate, as well as the effect on mineral content in erythrocyte cytosol.

The studies focusing on the effect of DHA on PTH, are limited and contradictory. First, available results showed lower values in the umbilical cord samples with respect to those found in adults and even in neonates at 2.5 months of life, results which are in agreement with those reported in the available scientific literature (Kovacs 2015; Sanz-Salvador et al. 2015). With regard to the effect of DHA supplementation, Kajarabille et al. (2018), (Kajarabille et al. 2018) found a significant increase in PTH during lactation in supplemented mothers and a lower concentration in neonates at 2.5 months of life. Other resorption biomarkers are cytokines, and in this sense, evidence suggests that pro-inflammatory biomarkers (IL-6 and TNF-α, among others) act on mesenchymal stem cells and osteoclast precursors enhancing bone resorption (Straburzynska-Lupa et al. 2013). Omega-3 LC PUFA supplementation shows a clear effect on these pro-inflammatory cytokines, decreasing the concentration of both cytokines in the mothers at the time of delivery and also decreasing IL-6 in the umbilical cord vein and TNF-α in umbilical cord artery at 2.5 months of life, findings that according to the mentioned above, could be beneficial for bone formation in neonate (Straburzynska-Lupa et al. 2013; Longo and Ward 2016).

The triad RANK/RANKL/osteoprotegerin (OPG) is a system of great importance in the regulation of bone metabolism and bone related pathophysiology (Mangano et al. 2013; Sanz-Salvador et al. 2015). While the binding of RANK to its ligand RANKL leads to bone resorption, OPG acts as an antagonist for RANK, avoiding the binding to the ligand, thus the binding of RANK to OPG inhibits bone resorption, and promotes bone formation (Mangano et al. 2013). In this way, Kajarabille et al. (2018), (Kajarabille et al. 2018) found significant differences in umbilical cord blood, reporting lower RANKL values in venous cord blood in mothers who were supplemented with omega-3 LC PUFA, as well as an increased OPG levels in arterial cord blood, which could be beneficial for the neonate, as bone resorption process decreases (Martin-Bautista et al. 2010). The results of Kajarabille et al. (2018), (Kajarabille et al. 2018) also showed higher OPN values in neonates, which highlights the high bone turnover rate in the neonate (Kovacs 2015). Kajarabille et al. (2018), (Kajarabille et al. 2018) showed higher concentrations of this biomarker in supplemented mothers at delivery, fact that could be related to the increased bone resorption in mother in order to supply more Ca to breast milk, as it has been described above. However, this cytokine has also a role as an inflammatory signal, and parturition leads to a significant inflammatory process which can promote an increase in OPN values as well (Straburzynska-Lupa et al. 2013). Regarding to OC, higher levels of this hormone have been found during lactation in mothers (Yoon et al. 2000). It has been observed the effect of the supplementation at delivery in mothers and at 2.5 months of neonate´s life, where an increase in OC has been found, which promotes neonate´s development and bone formation.

There are other hormones which have indirect effects such as ACTH, leptin or insulin. With regard to ACTH, we found significant differences in neonate´s umbilical cord vein samples, where supplemented group showed higher ACTH levels than the control group (Kajarabille et al. 2018). It has been reported that ACTH may stimulate osteoblast proliferation through specific receptors on these cells, which would enhance bone formation (Isales, Zaidi, and Blair 2010). On the other hand, Kajarabille et al., (2018), (Kajarabille et al. 2018) observed an increase of leptin in umbilical cord vein and artery blood in neonates whose mothers received the supplementation. According to biography, leptin has a double mechanism on bone metabolism, based on in vivo studies it appears that the peripheral effect which stimulates bone formation is the one that predominates, and therefore this could be beneficial for the neonate (Chen and Yang 2015). It has been also suggested that omega-3 fatty acids and leptin improve bone strength in mouse models (Mangano et al. 2013). Noteworthy, in spite of the leptin increase in the neonates of the supplemented mothers, Kajarabille et al. (2018), (Kajarabille et al. 2018) did not observed any changes in weight, fact that can be explained because as previously reported (Sominsky et al. 2017), short-term neonatal leptin antagonism did not reverse the excess body weight or hyperleptinemia in the neonatally overfed, suggesting factors other than leptin may also contribute to the phenotype and weight gain in the neonate. In addition, another hormone produced by osteocytes is fibroblast growth factor 23 (FGF23). FGF23 is best known for its role in various disorders of mineral metabolism. However, recent studies have found an association between circulating levels of FGF23, PTH, leptin and insulin sensitivity (Linossier et al. 2017).

Another hormone showing anabolic effects on bone is insulin due to a stimulating effect on insulin-like growth factor-1 (IGF1) synthesis (Hough et al. 2016). It has been reported an increase in umbilical cord artery and vein in neonates whose mothers received DHA supplementation. Other studies have shown DHA effects on insulin levels or insulin resistance (Calder 2016). High insulin concentrations in cord blood have been associated with appropriate weight gain during gestational age in infant (Mazaki-Tovi et al. 2005).

As important as the hormonal factors is the mineral content that is part of the hydroxyapatite. The mineral content in erythrocyte cytosol was also analyzed by Kajarabille et al. (2018), (Kajarabille et al. 2018). Ca and P are two minerals that together with bone homeostasis suffer significant changes during pregnancy and lactation due to the increased foetal requirements, particularly during the third trimester when rapid mineralization of the fetal skeleton occurs (Kovacs 2015; Sanz-Salvador et al. 2015). Omega-3 PUFA, and particularly DHA, improve Ca absorption, by modifying the composition of the intestinal membranes, thus reducing intestinal Ca loss (Griel et al. 2007). Kajarabille et al. (2018), (Kajarabille et al. 2018) showed an increase in the Ca concentration in mothers during lactation, which could help to cope with the increased requirements of maternal Ca during this period (Yoon et al. 2000) and in the neonates in umbilical cord vein and artery, helping to increase the supply of this mineral for adequate bone development (Kovacs 2015; Sanz-Salvador et al. 2015). P shows a similar trend with higher values in the supplemented mothers during delivery and lactation and in the umbilical cord artery, which could indicate a similar mechanism of omega-3 similar to the mentioned for Ca (Kajarabille et al. 2018). Other minerals such as Fe, Mg, Zn and Cu have also received some attention due to their role in bone turnover (Whiting et al. 2016). Neonates are particularly sensitive to imbalance in Fe metabolism (Cornock et al. 2013). The results of Kajarabille et al. (2018), (Kajarabille et al. 2018) showed that ω-3 LC PUFA during pregnancy and lactation increases Fe levels in the neonates. DHA has been shown to affect the expression of placental divalent metal transporters, as well as other Fe transporters (Diaz-Castro et al. 2015). With regard to Mg, data available showed significant differences between groups in mothers at postpartum and in umbilical cord vein in the neonates, where supplemented group had greater Mg concentration. Finally, Cu and Zn are necessary during gestation for proper foetal development (Mistry et al. 2014). The increase of Zn and Cu concentration per se, enables to strengthen the bone and also both minerals are essential for the proper functioning of immune system, as well as for the central nervous system (Mistry et al. 2014; Zhang et al. 2013). In addition, they also play a key role as cofactors of several antioxidant enzymes, such as Cu/Zn SOD (Zhang et al. 2013), which may help to explain the antioxidant effect observed by the DHA supplementation and could be another possible beneficial mechanism of action for bone formation in the neonates (Filaire and Toumi 2012). DHA supplementation increases Cu content in the mother during lactation and Zn in the neonate (umbilical cord artery and neonate at 2.5 months of life). In addition to the mechanisms previously discussed (Griel et al. 2007), other possible mechanisms through which supplementation with DHA could increase mineral content could be through inhibition of prostaglandin E2 (Kruger et al. 2010).

In summary, there are two stages of vital importance in bone development (gestation and lactation) and any modification in these periods would cause a greater risk of pathologies in later life. The ω-3 LC PUFA supplementation during pregnancy and lactation has beneficial effects on bone turnover in both mother and neonates, being the most noteworthy effect recorded in the neonate at birth and during first two months of postnatal life. In addition, ω-3 LC PUFA supplementation lead to an increase on mineral content in erythrocyte cytosol (especially Fe, Ca and P) in mothers and the neonates at delivery, assuring a suitable bone mineral recovery in mothers, as well as an adequate mineral content for the neonate, since the ossification process occurs rapidly during the first year of life.

REFERENCES

Bonewald, L. F. (2006). Mechanosensation and Transduction in Osteocytes. *BoneKEy osteovision*, 3 (10): 7-15. https://doi.org/10.1138/20060233.

Boyce, B. F., Yao, Z., and Xing, L. (2009). Osteoclasts have multiple roles in bone in addition to bone resorption. *Critical reviews in eukaryotic gene expression*, 19 (3): 171-80. https://doi.org/10.1615/critreveukargeneexpr.v19.i3.10.

Bozzetti, V., and Tagliabue, P. (2009). Metabolic Bone Disease in preterm newborn: an update on nutritional issues. *Italian journal of pediatrics*, 35 (1): 20. https://doi.org/10.1186/1824-7288-35-20.

Caetano-Lopes, J., Canhao, H., and Fonseca, J. E. (2007). Osteoblasts and bone formation. *Acta reumatologica portuguesa*, 32 (2): 103-10.

Calder, P. C. (2016). Docosahexaenoic Acid. *Annals of nutrition & metabolism*, 69 Suppl 1: 7-21. https://doi.org/10.1159/000448262.

Chan, G. M., Mileur, L., and Hansen, J. W. (1988). Calcium and phosphorus requirements in bone mineralization of preterm infants.

The Journal of pediatrics, 113 (1 Pt 2): 225-9. https://doi.org/10.1016/s0022-3476(88)80616-4.

Chen, X. X., and Yang, T. (2015). Roles of leptin in bone metabolism and bone diseases. *Journal of bone and mineral metabolism,* 33 (5): 474-85. https://doi.org/10.1007/s00774-014-0569-7.

Cornock, R., Gambling, L., Langley-Evans, S. C., McArdle, H. J., and McMullen, S. (2013). The effect of feeding a low iron diet prior to and during gestation on fetal and maternal iron homeostasis in two strains of rat. *Reproductive biology and endocrinology : RB&E,* 11: 32. https://doi.org/10.1186/1477-7827-11-32.

Diaz-Castro, J., Moreno-Fernández, J., Hijano, S., Kajarabille, N., Pulido-Moran, M., Latunde-Dada, G. O., Hurtado, J. A., Peña, M., Peña-Quintana, L., Lara-Villoslada, F., and Ochoa, J. J. (2015). DHA supplementation: A nutritional strategy to improve prenatal Fe homeostasis and prevent birth outcomes related with Fe-deficiency. *Journal of Functional Foods,* 19: 385-393. https://doi.org/https://doi.org/10.1016/j.jff.2015.09.051.

Filaire, E., and Toumi, H. (2012). Reactive oxygen species and exercise on bone metabolism: friend or enemy? *Joint, bone, spine: revue du rhumatisme,* 79 (4): 341-6. https://doi.org/10.1016/j.jbspin.2012.03.007.

Frost, H. M. (1997). On our age-related bone loss: insights from a new paradigm. *Journal of bone and mineral research: the official journal of the American Society for Bone and Mineral Research,* 12 (10): 1539-46. https://doi.org/10.1359/jbmr.1997.12.10.1539.

Gertner, J. M., Coustan, D. R., Kliger, A. S., Mallette, L. E., Ravin, N., and Broadus, A. E. (1986). Pregnancy as state of physiologic absorptive hypercalciuria. *The American journal of medicine,* 81 (3): 451-6. https://doi.org/10.1016/0002-9343(86)90298-6.

Glerean, M., and Plantalech, L. (2000). [Osteoporosis in pregnancy and lactation]. *Medicina,* 60 (6): 973-81.

Griel, A. E., Kris-Etherton, P. M., Hilpert, K. F., Zhao, G., West, S. G., and Corwin, R. L. (2007). An increase in dietary n-3 fatty acids decreases a marker of bone resorption in humans. *Nutrition journal*, 6: 2. https://doi.org/10.1186/1475-2891-6-2.

Harrison, C. M., and Gibson, A. T. (2013). Osteopenia in preterm infants. *Archives of disease in childhood. Fetal and neonatal edition*, 98 (3): F272-5. https://doi.org/10.1136/archdischild-2011-301025.

Hough, F. S., Pierroz, D. D., Cooper, C., and Ferrari, S. L. (2016). Mechanisms In Endocrinology: Mechanisms and evaluation of bone fragility in type 1 diabetes mellitus. *European journal of endocrinology*, 174 (4): R127-38. https://doi.org/10.1530/eje-15-0820.

Huddleston, J. F., Sanchez-Ramos, L., and Huddleston, K. W. (2003). Acute management of preterm labor. *Clinics in perinatology*, 30 (4): 803-24, vii. https://doi.org/10.1016/s0095-5108(03)00114-3.

Indumati, V., Patil, Vidya S., and Jailkhani, Rama. (2007). Hospital based preliminary study on osteoporosis in postmenopausal women. *Indian J Clin Biochem*, 22 (2): 96-100. https://doi.org/10.1007/BF02913323.

Isales, C. M., Zaidi, M., and Blair, H. C. (2010). ACTH is a novel regulator of bone mass. *Annals of the New York Academy of Sciences*, 1192: 110-6. https://doi.org/10.1111/j.1749-6632.2009.05231.x.

Jain, S., and Cheng, J. (2006). Emergency department visits and rehospitalizations in late preterm infants. *Clinics in perinatology*, 33 (4): 935-45; abstract xi. https://doi.org/10.1016/j.clp.2006.09.007.

Kajarabille, N., Peña, M., Díaz-Castro, J., Hurtado, J. A., Peña-Quintana, L., Iznaola, C., Rodríguez-Santana, Y., Martin-Alvarez, E., López-Frias, M., Lara-Villoslada, F., and Ochoa, J. J. (2018). Omega-3 LCPUFA supplementation improves neonatal and maternal bone turnover: A randomized controlled trial. *Journal of Functional Foods*, 46: 167-174. https://doi.org/https://doi.org/10.1016/j.jff.2018.04.065.

Kovacs, C. S. (2011). Bone development in the fetus and neonate: role of the calciotropic hormones. *Current osteoporosis reports*, 9 (4): 274-83. https://doi.org/10.1007/s11914-011-0073-0.

Kovacs, C. S. (2014). Bone metabolism in the fetus and neonate. *Pediatric nephrology (Berlin, Germany)*, 29 (5): 793-803. https://doi.org/10.1007/s00467-013-2461-4.

Kovacs, C. S. (2015). Calcium, phosphorus, and bone metabolism in the fetus and newborn. *Early human development,* 91 (11): 623-8. https://doi.org/10.1016/j.earlhumdev.2015.08.007.

Kruger, M. C., Coetzee, M., Haag, M., and Weiler, H. (2010). Long-chain polyunsaturated fatty acids: selected mechanisms of action on bone. *Progress in lipid research,* 49 (4): 438-49. https://doi.org/10.1016/j.plipres.2010.06.002.

Linossier, Marie-Thérèse, Amirova, Liubov E., Thomas, Mireille, Normand, Myriam, Bareille, Marie-Pierre, Gauquelin-Koch, Guillemette, Beck, Arnaud, Costes-Salon, Marie-Claude, Bonneau, Christine, Gharib, Claude, Custaud, Marc-Antoine, and Vico, Laurence. (2017). Effects of short-term dry immersion on bone remodeling markers, insulin and adipokines. *PLOS ONE,* 12 (8): e0182970. https://doi.org/10.1371/journal.pone.0182970.

Longo, A. B., and Ward, W. E. (2016). PUFAs, Bone Mineral Density, and Fragility Fracture: Findings from Human Studies. *Advances in nutrition (Bethesda, Md.),* 7 (2): 299-312. https://doi.org/10.3945/an.115.009472.

Maness, S. B., and Buhi, E. R. (2016). Associations Between Social Determinants of Health and Pregnancy Among Young People: A Systematic Review of Research Published During the Past 25 Years. *Public health reports* (Washington, D.C.: 1974), 131 (1): 86 99. https://doi.org/10.1177/003335491613100115.

Mangano, K. M., Sahni, S., Kerstetter, J. E., Kenny, A. M., and Hannan, M. T. (2013). Polyunsaturated fatty acids and their relation with bone and muscle health in adults. *Current osteoporosis reports,* 11 (3): 203-12. https://doi.org/10.1007/s11914-013-0149-0.

Martin-Bautista, E., Munoz-Torres, M., Fonolla, J., Quesada, M., Poyatos, A., and Lopez-Huertas, E. (2010). Improvement of bone formation biomarkers after 1-year consumption with milk fortified with eicosapentaenoic acid, docosahexaenoic acid, oleic acid, and selected vitamins. *Nutrition research (New York, N.Y.),* 30 (5): 320-6. https://doi.org/10.1016/j.nutres.2010.05.007.

Mazaki-Tovi, S., Kanety, H., Pariente, C., Hemi, R., Schiff, E., and Sivan, E. (2005). Cord blood adiponectin in large-for-gestational age newborns. *American journal of obstetrics and gynecology*, 193 (3 Pt 2): 1238-42. https://doi.org/10.1016/j.ajog.2005.05.049.

Mistry, H. D., Kurlak, L. O., Young, S. D., Briley, A. L., Pipkin, F. B., Baker, P. N., and Poston, L. (2014). Maternal selenium, copper and zinc concentrations in pregnancy associated with small-for-gestational-age infants. *Maternal & child nutrition*, 10 (3): 327-34. https://doi.org/10.1111/j.1740-8709.2012.00430.x.

Poulsen, R. C., Moughan, P. J., and Kruger, M. C. (2007). Long-chain polyunsaturated fatty acids and the regulation of bone metabolism. *Experimental biology and medicine (Maywood, N.J.)*, 232 (10): 1275-88. https://doi.org/10.3181/0704-mr-100.

Rustico, S. E., Calabria, A. C., and Garber, S. J. (2014). Metabolic bone disease of prematurity. *Journal of clinical & translational endocrinology*, 1 (3): 85-91. https://doi.org/10.1016/j.jcte.2014.06.004.

Sanz-Salvador, L., Garcia-Perez, M. A., Tarin, J. J., and Cano, A. (2015). Bone metabolic changes during pregnancy: a period of vulnerability to osteoporosis and fracture. *European journal of endocrinology*, 172 (2): R53-65. https://doi.org/10.1530/eje-14-0424.

Smith, Everett L., and Clark, Wendy D. (2005). Cellular Control of Bone Response to Physical Activity. *Topics in Geriatric Rehabilitation*, 21 (1): 77-87. https://journals.lww.com/topicsingeriatricrehabilitation/Fulltext/2005/01000/Cellular_Control_of_Bone_Response_to_Physical.9.aspx.

Sominsky, L., Ziko, I., Nguyen, T. X., Quach, J., and Spencer, S. J. (2017). Hypothalamic effects of neonatal diet: reversible and only partially leptin dependent. *The Journal of endocrinology*, 234 (1): 41-56. https://doi.org/10.1530/joe-16-0631.

Straburzynska-Lupa, A., Nowak, A., Romanowski, W., Korman, P., and Pilaczynska-Szczesniak, L. (2013). A study of the link between bone turnover markers and bone mineral density with inflammation and body mass in postmenopausal women with active rheumatoid arthritis.

Journal of bone and mineral metabolism, 31 (2): 169-76. https://doi.org/10.1007/s00774-012-0400-2.

Tucker, J., and McGuire, W. (2004). Epidemiology of preterm birth. *BMJ (Clinical research ed.)*, 329 (7467): 675-8. https://doi.org/10.1136/bmj.329.7467.675.

Wang, M. L., Dorer, D. J., Fleming, M. P., and Catlin, E. A. (2004). Clinical outcomes of near-term infants. *Pediatrics*, 114 (2): 372-6. https://doi.org/10.1542/peds.114.2.372.

Whiting, S. J., Kohrt, W. M., Warren, M. P., Kraenzlin, M. I., and Bonjour, J. P. (2016). Food fortification for bone health in adulthood: a scoping review. *European journal of clinical nutrition*, 70 (10): 1099-1105. https://doi.org/10.1038/ejcn.2016.42.

WHO. (2012). Born Too Soon. Global Action Report on Premature Births. *World Health Organization*.

Yoon, B. K., Lee, J. W., Choi, D. S., Roh, C. R., and Lee, J. H. (2000). Changes in biochemical bone markers during pregnancy and puerperium. *J Korean Med Sci*, 15 (2): 189-193. https://doi.org/10.3346/jkms.2000.15.2.189.
https://www.ncbi.nlm.nih.gov/pubmed/10803696.

Yoshida, K., Oida, H., Kobayashi, T., Maruyama, T., Tanaka, M., Katayama, T., Yamaguchi, K., Segi, E., Tsuboyama, T., Matsushita, M., Ito, K., Ito, Y., Sugimoto, Y., Ushikubi, F., Ohuchida, S., Kondo, K., Nakamura, T., and Narumiya, S. (2002). Stimulation of bone formation and prevention of bone loss by prostaglandin E EP4 receptor activation. *Proceedings of the National Academy of Sciences of the United States of America*, 99 (7): 4580-5. https://doi.org/10.1073/pnas.062053399.

Zhang, Z., Yuan, E., Liu, J., Lou, X., Jia, L., Li, X., and Zhang, L. (2013). Gestational age-specific reference intervals for blood copper, zinc, calcium, magnesium, iron, lead, and cadmium during normal pregnancy. *Clinical biochemistry*, 46 (9): 777-80. https://doi.org/10.1016/j.clinbiochem.2013.03.004.

In: Preterm Birth
Editors: A. Malik and A. Baarda
ISBN: 978-1-53618-298-9
© 2020 Nova Science Publishers, Inc.

Chapter 4

MATERNAL PERIODONTAL DISEASE AND ADVERSE PREGNANCY OUTCOMES: THE CURRENT STAND

Jananni Muthu[1,*]
and Sivaramakrishnan Muthanandam[2]
[1]Department of Periodontology,
[2]Department of Oral Pathology and Microbiology,
Indira Gandhi Institute of Dental sciences,
Sri Balaji Vidyapeeth (Deemed to be) University, Pondicherry, India

ABSTRACT

Periodontitis is a multifactorial chronic inflammatory disease of the supporting structures of the tooth, which when untreated can result in loss of function of the teeth and eventually tooth loss. The primary etiology for periodontal disease is the bacterial pathogens that evoke a host inflammatory response. The host bacterial interaction is not only localized to the oral cavity but also evokes systemic response elsewhere

---

* Corresponding Author's E-mail: jannpearl@gmail.com.

in the body. In the few past decades chronic periodontal disease has been linked to various systemic diseases like cardiovascular diseases, diabetes mellitus, respiratory illnesses, renal diseases and adverse pregnancy outcomes, leading to the emergence of a new branch of periodontology known as periodontal medicine.

Adverse pregnancy outcomes represent an important health issue which affects not only the infant but also the mother. There is evidence that adverse pregnancy outcomes are correlated with intra-uterine infections and increased local and systemic inflammatory markers. Periodontitis being a chronic inflammatory disease might contribute to this systemic inflammation. The most common adverse pregnancy outcomes that have been associated with chronic periodontal disease are premature rupture of membranes and preterm birth, low birth weight, and preeclampsia. Research in the past few years have established periodontal disease as a risk factor for adverse pregnancy outcomes and studies have also proved that treatment of periodontal disease reduced the risk for adverse pregnancy outcomes. This paper aims in exploring the mechanisms that link periodontitis with adverse pregnancy outcomes and also presents a comprehensive critical review of the current scientific stand regarding this relationship.

INTRODUCTION

In the past few decades research in the field of periodontology has been focused on the two-way relationship in which periodontal disease in an individual may be a powerful influence on an individual's systemic health or disease as well as the more customarily understood role that systemic disease may have in influencing an individual's periodontal health or disease. This has led to the emergence of a new branch of periodontology known as periodontal medicine, which integrates periodontology and internal medicine [1]. The American Academy of Periodontology has rightly stated that "Periodontal bacteria can enter the bloodstream and travel to major organs and begin new infections. Evidence suggesting that this process may contribute to the development of heart disease; increase the risk of stroke; increase a woman's risk of delivering a preterm low-birth weight baby; and pose a serious threat to people whose health is compromised by diabetes mellitus, respiratory disease or osteoporosis" [1].

ADVERSE PREGNANCY OUTCOMES

Pregnancy outcomes refer to life events that occur to the newborn infant from the age of viability (28 weeks) to the first week of life. Adverse pregnancy outcomes are those pregnancy outcomes other than normal live birth which majorly include preterm birth, stillbirth and low birth weight, which are the major causes of neonatal morbidity, mortality and long term physical and psychological problems [2]. Among these, pre term and low birth weight are the most common adverse pregnancy outcomes in developing counties and are considered to be the most relevant biological determinants of newborn infant's survival [3]. It has been estimated that 12% of babies are born prematurely, 8% with low birth weight, and 3% have major birth defects [4].

The following are the most studied risk factors for PT/LBW infant deliveries: maternal age (>34yrs and <17yrs), improper pre natal care, smoking, alcohol or drug use during pregnancy, hypertension, adverse behaviors, nutritional status, diabetes, uterine contractions and cervical length and infections [5, 6, 7].

INFLUENCE OF PREGNANCY ON ORAL HEALTH

As early as in 1800 gingival changes during pregnancy have been identified. Like other systemic conditions, pregnancy per se does not cause gingival diseases [8, 9]. Gingival disease, namely pregnancy gingivitis, is the result of accentuated response to the dental plaque caused by the hormonal changes induced by the pregnant state. No notable change in the gingiva can happen in pregnant women without plaque [10, 11]. The severity of gingivitis increases during second or third month of pregnancy and becomes more severe by the eighth month [10]. The accentuation of gingivitis peaks at this time due to the fact that during the first trimester there is over production of gonadotropins and during the third trimester the estrogen and progesterone levels are highest.

This is attributed to host bacterial interplay that leads to gingival inflammation. *P. intermedia*, a potential periodontal pathogen, is found in increased numbers during pregnancy. It is owed to the fact that during pregnancy, the increased levels of progesterone is utilized by the bacteria as source of nutrient [12]. Moreover the hormone also increases the dilation and tortuosity of the gingival capillaries. The capillary walls become engorged, thin and ulcerated. This eventually results in edema and increased gingival bleeding [13, 14].

In some cases the inflamed gingiva present as a discrete tumor-like mass known as pregnancy tumor. This is a localized gingival enlargement due to non-specific proliferative inflammation [15]. This is a benign mass and if it interferes with occlusion or is painful due to ulceration, total excision can be considered.

Does Periodontal Disease Pose a Systemic Threat?

In the early 18th century physicians emerged with a new concept of "The Focal Infection Theory," according to which, a localized infection in one part of the body can disseminate the infectious agent or toxic products and can significantly influence events elsewhere in the body. Periodontal disease is by far the most common oral infection caused by bacteria due to accumulation of dental plaque. The bacteria initiates a cascade of reactions that leads to destruction of supporting structures of the tooth eventually leading to tooth mobility and loss. This localized infection in the oral cavity can pose a systemic threat in three ways [16]:

1. Subgingival biofilm – accumulates bacteria and provides an easy access to general circulation.
2. Shared risk factors - Age, ethnicity, smoking, stress etc are common to periodontal disease as well as other systemic diseases.

3. Periodontium – cytokine reservoir – Periodontal pathogens secrete wide range of cytokines that exert a generalized systemic effect.

PERIODONTAL PATHOGENS AND SYSTEMIC INFECTION

Periodontal pathogens' three important properties that enable them to exert their effect in other systems of the body:

1. The ability to colonize
2. The ability to elude the host's defense mechanisms
3. The ability to produce substances leading directly to tissue destruction.

Among the various periodontal pathogens, the most studied are the *Porphyromonas gingivalis and Aggrigatebacter actinomycetemcommitans.* These bacteria possess a tissue invading property, thus penetrating the epithelial cells, entering into the connective tissue and evoking a host immune response [17]. Bacterial LPS induce numerous host defence cells, including fibroblasts, to produce a variety of cytokines, matrix metalloproteinases and other pro inflammatory mediators, including arachidonic acid metabolites. IL-1, IL-6, IL-8, TNF-a, and PGE2 are the common pro inflammatory mediators whose levels are increased in periodontal infection. Interleukin 1 is a proinflammatory cytokine which promotes the entry of inflammatory cells into the infection site and stimulates the release of eicosanoids. Interleukin 6 stimulates the proliferation of plasma cells, thus generating secondary antibody production. High levels of IL-6 are found in inflamed tissues. PGE2 is a vasoactive eicosanoid produced by monocytes and fibroblasts.

Placenta can never be sterile and bacterial infiltration of the placenta has been extensively studied. Variations in placental microbiome is reported to be associated with pregnancy outcomes. Intra amniotic infection has been strongly associated with preterm birth but the source of infections is less known [18]. Though ascending infection from vagina is a possibility, hematogenous source of infection should also be probed. This concept is proved by detection of oral microorganisms in the placenta. When this bacteria are from a periodontal infection, they have more virulence and they modulate an inflammatory response that results in adverse pregnancy outcomes [19].

Studies have also found that periodontal pathogens are more prevalent in the placentas of women with periodontal disease [20]. A variety of key periodontal pathogens have been identified in the placenta of women with periodontitis, including *P. gingivalis* and *F. nucleatum* [21, 22]. *F. nucleatum* plays a role in a host of adverse pregnancy outcomes, including hypertensive disorders, preterm birth, low birth weight, chorioamnionitis, miscarriage, stillbirth, and early onset neonatal sepsis [23].

MECHANISM LINKING PERIODONTAL INFECTION AND ADVERSE PREGNANCY OUTCOMES

Bacterial Vaginosis

This is a common infectious disorder of the female reproductive tract. When the lactobacilli, a commensal in the vaginal tract, is replaced by species like *Gardenella vaginalis, peptostrptococcus, porphyromonas* etc, it leads to bacterial vaginosis [24]. Bacterial vaginosis has been a documented risk factor for adverse pregnancy outcomes. One important oral periodontal pathogen associated with bacterial vaginosis is *F. nucleatum,* which has been isolated in vaginal flora and is more prevalent in women with pre-term labor. Primary mechanism that causes APO is the ascending infection from the vagina and endocervix [25]. This infection injures the tissue wall as well as induces the over production of inflammatory mediators to labor inducing levels. Indirect mechanism may be due to bacterial infection of the chorioamnion and extra placental membranes leading to PROM and premature delivery [26].

Role of Periodontitis

In various pregnancy related pathologies, systemic inflammation has been found to have a major role. Though the pathology of adverse pregnancy outcomes is thought to be multifactorial, like stress, immune mediated processes, infection, hemorrhage, uteroplacental ischemia etc., development of pro inflammatory conditions is considered as a common pathway that unifies all the multiple risk factors [27, 28]. Constant chronic up regulation of pro inflammatory cytokines at the fetomaternal interface will eventually lead to membrane weakening, early membrane rupture, and uterine contraction initiation, resulting in adverse pregnancy outcomes [29].

Periodontal disease, as a remote Gram negative infection, may have the potential to affect pregnancy outcome. The host's inflammatory response to the periodontal infection appears to be the critical determinant resulting in adverse pregnancy outcomes. In the case of periodontal infection, during pregnancy, the vascular supply and the vascular permeability to the periodontium increases [30]. With this high bacterial load and increased permeability of the vessels, even simple day to day manipulations like tooth brushing, chewing food etc can result in hematogenous spread of oral bacteria and inflammatory mediators to the fetal–maternal unit [31].

Periodontitis causes adverse pregnancy outcomes through two different mechanisms [32].

1. Increased levels of pro inflammatory mediators are present at the site of periodontal infection and they can be transported to amniotic fluid via maternal circulation?
2. The lipopolysaccharide layer of periodontal pathogens, especially *P. gingivalis* and *a. actinomycetemcommitans,* increases the placental levels of TNF and PGE2. This enteric endotoxin also induces placental necrosis which results in even spontaneous abortions. Other complications might include fetal organ damage and malformations [33].

Another mechanism that has been proposed is that related to Toll like receptors. TLR are trans membrane proteins which when activated by bacterial LPS, signals the nucleus through the cytoplasm to encode genes for secretion of cytokines. This LPS activation of TLR is seen even in placenta where it signals for over production of cytokines, eventually leading to adverse pregnancy outcomes [34].

Mechanism of Overlapping Genetic Substrates – Epigenetic Concept

Genes associated with dampening of the host immune responses predispose to pre-term. Inflammatory genes, which are the genes that influence the response to infection, are also found to influence the function of placenta and uterus. Thus these genes directly influence the pregnancy outcomes [35]. Mutations in the following genes are associated with activation of inflammasomes and also have been implicated in pre-term premature rupture of membranes: CARD6, DEFB1, MBL2, NLRP10, NOD2, and possibly FUT2 [36]. These overlapping genetic substrates predispose to spontaneous preterm birth and known inflammatory conditions, e.g., inflammatory bowel disease and periodontal disease [37].

WHAT DOES THE EVIDENCE POINT TO? [38]

Analysis of case-control, cross sectional and prospective studies:

Maternal Periodontitis and Low Birth Weight

Jacob & Nath, 2014 [39]; Reza Karimi et al., 2015 [40]; Gomes-Filho et al., 2016 [41], Tellapragada et al., 2016 [42]; Lohana et al., 2017 [43] reported significant association between LBW and maternal periodontitis.

Abati et al., 2013 [44] did not find any correlation between maternal periodontitis and LBW.

Maternal Periodontitis and Preterm Birth

Guimarães et al., 2010 [45]; Giannella et al., 2011 [46]; Piscoya et al., 2012 [47]., Macedo et al., 2014 [48] Martínez de Tejada et al., 2012 [49] reported significant association whereas few authors like Nabet et al., 2010 [50]; Iwanaga et al., 2011 [51] Bulut et al., 2014 [52] Jain et al., 2016 [53] did not find any correlation between the two.

Maternal Periodontitis and Pre-Eclampsia

Abati et al., (2013) [44], Chaparro et al., (2013) [54] Hirano et al., (2012) [55] did not find any correlation between the two entities. Moura da Silva et al., 2012 [56]; Ide and Papapanou (2013) [57] found a statistically significant relation between the two.

On analyzing the available literature evidence, considering low birth weight infants, there might be an association with periodontitis. The evidence on preterm birth would suggest a higher tendency for periodontitis in women who deliver preterm. Pre-eclampsia appeared to be associated with periodontitis.

Analysis of Systematic Reviews and Meta-Analysis

Vettore MV et al., 2006 [58], reported no significant association between maternal periodontal disease and adverse pregnancy outcomes. Corbella S et al., 2018 [59], reported a low but existing association between periodontal disease and adverse pregnancy outcomes. Vivares Ba et al., 2018 [60] reported that there is a relationship between clinical periodontal disease and adverse birth outcomes. Teshome A et al., [61], concluded that periodontal disease may be one of the possible risk factors for preterm low birth weight infants. Ide et al., 2013 [57] reported that maternal periodontitis is modestly but independently associated with adverse pregnancy outcomes. Correder ED et al., [62], and Sayfer IF et al., 2019 [63] concluded that pregnant mothers with periodontitis double the risk of preterm birth.

Daalderop LA 2018 [64], in an overview of systematic reviews reported that pregnant women with periodontal disease are at increased risk of developing preeclampsia and delivering a preterm and/or LBW baby. The authors also stated that "the association between periodontal disease and various common and severe adverse pregnancy outcomes is now sufficiently established for the field to start moving beyond conducting additional primary epidemiologic studies and systematic reviews in this area. They also suggested that now the focus should shift on the mechanism and development of preventive treatment modalities and targeted therapies.

Corbella A et al., 2012 [65] found no clear evidence that periodontal disease is a major risk factor for adverse pregnancy outcomes, although it may exert a minor effect. Non-surgical periodontal therapy is safe during pregnancy, but the current study found no evidence of its efficacy in reducing the incidence of preterm birth or low birth weight.

EFFECT OF PERIODONTAL TREATMENT ON ADVERSE PREGNANCY OUTCOMES

Kim JA et al., [66], in his systematic review and meta-analysis, indicates statistically significant effect in reducing risk of preterm birth for SRP in pregnant women with periodontitis for groups with high risks of preterm birth only. Oliveria P et al., 2010 [67] in a systematic review concluded that non-surgical periodontal treatment in pregnant women decreased the risk for pregnancy outcomes. Schwenicke F et al., 2015 [68] suggested that providing periodontal treatment to pregnant women could potentially reduce the risks of perinatal outcomes, especially in mothers with high risks. Bi et al., 2019 [69] found that periodontal treatment during pregnancy reduces the risks of perinatal mortality and preterm birth, and improves birth weight.

Results from Fogacci et al., [70] do not support the hypothesis that periodontal therapy reduces preterm birth and LBW indices. Uppal A et al., 2010 [71] reported that pooled results from the highest-quality RCTs do not support the hypothesis of a reduction of PTB or LBW in women who are treated for periodontal disease during pregnancy. Rosa M et al., 2010 [72] summarized that primary periodontal care during pregnancy cannot be considered an efficient way of reducing the incidence of preterm birth. Corbella A et al., 2012 [65] found no evidence of its efficacy in reducing the incidence of preterm birth or low birth weight.

On analyzing literature evidence for the treatment outcomes, there seems to be a wide disparity in results. But considering the association between the periodontal diseases and adverse pregnancy outcomes, dental interventions can be recommended as preventive therapy for preterm birth.

CONCLUSION

There appears to be a two-way relationship between periodontal conditions and the state of pregnancy. The fact that pregnancy causes a marked change in the gingival health is well documented and accepted by the scientific community. When considering the other way relation, i.e., periodontal diseases resulting in adverse pregnancy outcomes, the evidence is moderate although some studies claim that it is an independent risk factor for pre term low birth. On analyzing the interventional studies as proof of causation, results of existing intervention studies are mixed, with some showing a beneficial effect and others finding no benefit. Nevertheless, awareness among general medical practitioners of this link between periodontal infection and low term birth weight will improve pregnancy outcomes.

REFERENCES

[1] American Academy of Periodontology. (2008). *Oral Health Information for the Public: Mouth Body Connection.* www.perio.org/consumer/mbc.top2.htm. Accessed Jan 16.
[2] Vibal chaiba B., (2014). Determinants of adverse pregnancy outcomes in Mutare district clinics. *Inter J Obstetrics Gynaeco,* 7: 62 – 75.
[3] Baskaradoss, J. K., Geevarghese, A., Al Dosari, A. (2012). Causes of adverse pregnancy outcomes and the role of maternal periodontal status - a review of the literature. *The open dentistry journal,* 6: 79–84.
[4] Althabe, F., Bhutta, Z., Blencowe, H., Chandramouli, V., Chou D., et al., (2012). In *Born too soon: The global action report on preterm birth,* Edited by Christopher Howson MK, Joy L. Geneva, Switzerland: WHO.
[5] Verkerk, P. H., van Noord-Zaadstra, B. M., Florey, C. D., de Jonge, G. A., Verloove-Vanhorick, S. P. (1993). The effect of moderate maternal alcohol consumption on birth weight and gestational age in a low risk population. *Early Hum Dev,* 32: 121–9.
[6] Copper, R. L., Goldenberg, R. L, Das, A., et al., (1996). The preterm prediction study: maternal stress is associated with spontaneous preterm birth at less than thirty-five weeks' gestation. National Institute of Child Health and Human Development Maternal-Fetal Medicine Units Network. *Am J Obstet Gynecol,* 175(5): 1286–92.
[7] Romero, B. C., Chiquito, C. S., Elejalde, L. E., Bernardoni, C. B. (2002). Relationship between periodontal disease in pregnant women and the nutritional condition of their newborns. *J Periodontol,* 73: 1177–83.
[8] Biro. (1898). Studies regarding influence of pregnancy on caries. *Viertel – jahschr zahnheilk,* 14: 7 – 54.
[9] Pinard. (1877). Gingivitis in pregnancy. *Dent register,* 31: 158.
[10] Loe. (1965). Periodontal changes in pregnancy. *J periodontal,* 3: 209 – 214.

[11] Maier, A. W., Orban, B. (1949). Gingivitis in pregnancy. *Oral Surg Oral Med Oral Pathol*, 2: 334-73.
[12] Kornman, K. S., Loesche, W. J. (1980). The subgingival microflora during pregnancy. *J Periodontal Res*, 15: 111 - 122.
[13] Mohammad, A., Waterhouse, J. P., Friederici, H. H. (1974). The micro vasculature of rat gingiva as affected by progesterone: an ultra structural study. *J Periodontol*, 45: 50.
[14] O'Leary, T., Shannaon, L., Prigmore, J. R. (1962). Clinical and systematic findings in periodontal disease. *J Periodontal*, 32: 243.
[15] Ziskin, D., Blackberg, S. N., Stout, A. (1933). The gingiva during pregnancy: an experimental study and histopathological interpretation. *Surg Gynecol Obstet*, 57: 1930 – 37.
[16] Page, R. C. (1998). The pathobiology of periodontal diseases may affect systemic diseases: inversion of a paradigm. *Ann. Periodontol*, 3: 108-120.
[17] Lin, D., Smith, M. A., Champagne, C., Elter, J., Beck, J., Offenbacher, S., (2003). Porphyromonas gingivalis infection during pregnancy increases maternal tumor necrosis factor alpha, suppresses maternal interleukin-10, and enhances fetal growth restriction and resorption in mice. *Infect Immunol*, 71(9): 5156-5162.
[18] Cobb, C. M., Kelly, P. J., Williams, K. B., Babbar, S., Angolkar, M., Derman, R. J. (2017). The oral microbiome and adverse pregnancy outcomes. *Int J Womens Health*, 9: 551–9.
[19] Gomez-Arango, L. F., Barrett, H. L., McIntyre, H. D., Callaway, L. K., Morrison, M., Nitert, M. D. (2017). Contributions of the maternal oral and gut microbiome to placental microbial colonization in overweight and obese pregnant women. *Sci Rep*, 7: 2860.
[20] Blanc, V., O'Valle, F., Pozo, E., Puertas, A., León, R., Mesa, F. (2015). Oral bacteria in placental tissues: increased molecular detection in pregnant periodontitis patients. *Oral Dis*, 21: 905–12.
[21] Vander Haar, E. L., So, J., Gyamfi-Bannerman, C., Han, YW. (2018). Fusobacterium nucleatum and adverse pregnancy outcomes: epidemiological and mechanistic evidence. *Anaerobe*, 50:55–9.

[22] Prince, A. L., Ma, J., Kannan, P. S., Alvarez, M., Gisslen, T., Harris, R. A., et al., (2016). The placental membrane microbiome is altered among subjects with spontaneous preterm birth with and without chorioamnionitis. *Am J Obstet Gynecol*, 214: 627.

[23] Fischer, L. A., Demerath, E., Bittner-Eddy, P., Costalonga, M., Bittner- Eddy, P., Costalonga, M., et al., (2019). Placental colonization with periodontal pathogens: the potential missing link. *Am J Obstet Gynecol*, 221: 383–92.

[24] Grossi, S. G., Mealy, B. L., Rose, L. F. (2004). Effect of periodontal infection on systemic health. In Rose LF, Mealy BL, Genco RJ, Cohen DW, editors: *Periodontics: Medicine, Surgery and Implants*, St Louis, Elsiever.

[25] Hill, G. B. (1998). Preterm birth associated with genital and possibly oral micoflora. *Ann Periodontol*, 3: 222 – 232.

[26] Williams, C., Davenport, E., Sterne, J et al., (2000). Mechanisms of risk in pre-term infants. *Periodontology 2000*, 23: 142 – 150.

[27] Romero, R., Espinoza, J., Gonc¸alves, L. F., Kusanovic, J. P., Friel, L. A., Nien, J. K., (2006). Inflammation in preterm and term labour and delivery. *Semin Fetal Neonatal Med*, 11(5): 317-326.

[28] Romero, R., Gomez, R., Galasso, M., et al., (1994). Macrophage inflammatory protein-1 alpha in term and preterm parturition: effect of microbial invasion of the amniotic cavity. *Am J Reprod Immuno*, 32(2): 108-113.

[29] Shoji, T., Yoshida, S., Mitsunari, M., et al., 2007. Involvement of p38 MAP kinase in lipopolysaccharide-induced production of pro- and anti-inflammatory cytokines and prostaglandin E(2) in human choriodecidua. *J Reprod Immunol*, 75(2): 82-90.

[30] Offenbacher, S., Jared, H. L., O'Reilly, P. G., et al., (1998). Potential pathogenic mechanisms of periodontitis associated pregnancy complications. *Ann Periodontol*, 3: 233–50.

[31] Klebanoff, M., Searle, K. (2006). The role of inflammation in preterm birth – focus on periodontitis. *Br J Obstet Gynaecol*, 8: 113 – 119.

[32] Dortbudak, O., Eberhardt, R., Ulm, M., Persson, G. R., (2005). Periodontitis, a marker of risk in pregnancy for preterm birth. *J Clin Periodontol,* 32(1): 45-52.

[33] Haesaert, B., Ornoy, A,. (1986). Transplacental effects of endotoxemia on fetal mouse brain, bone and placental tissue. *Pedriatr Pathol,* 5: 167-181.

[34] Akira S,. (2003). Toll-like receptor signaling. *J Biol Chem,* 278: 38105-38108.

[35] Hallman, M., Haapalainen, A., Huusko, J. M., Karjalainen, M. K., Zhang, G., Muglia, L. J., et al., (2019). Spontaneous premature birth as a target of genomic research. *Pediatr Res,* 85: 422–31.

[36] Modi, B. P., Teves, M. E., Pearson, L. N., Parikh, H. I., Haymond-Thornburg, H., Tucker, J. L., et al., (2017). Mutations in fetal genes involved in innate immunity and host defense against microbes increase risk of preterm premature rupture of membranes (PPROM). *Mol Genet Genomic Med,* 5: 720–9.

[37] Strauss, J. F., Romero, R., Gomez-Lopez, N., Haymond-Thornburg, H., Modi, B. P., Teves, M. E, et al., (2018). Spontaneous preterm birth: advances toward the discovery of genetic predisposition. *Am J Obstet Gynecol,*; 218: 294–314.e2.

[38] Petrini, M., Gürsoy, M., Gennai, S., Graziani, F,. (2017). Biological mechanisms between periodontal diseases and pregnancy complications: a systematic review and meta-analysis of epidemiological association between adverse pregnancy outcomes and periodontitis – an update of the review by Ide & Papapanou (2013). Oral health and pregnancy, *European federation of periodontology,* 1- 39.

[39] Jacob, P. S. & Nath, S. (2014). Periodontitis among poor rural Indian mothers increases the risk of low birth weight babies: a hospital-based case control study. *Journal of Periodontal & Implant Science,* 44:85-93.

[40] Reza, Karimi, M., Hamissi, J. H., Naeini, S. R. & Karimi, M. (2015). The relationship between maternal periodontal status of and preterm

and low birth weight infants in Iran: A case control study. *Global Journal of Health Science*, 8: 184-188.

[41] Gomes-Filho, I. S., Pereira, E. C., Cruz, S. S., Adan, L. F. F., Vianna, M. P., Passos-Soares, J. S., et al., (2016). Relationship among mothers' glycemic level, periodontitis, and birth weight. *Journal of Periodontology*, 7: 238-247.

[42] Tellapragada, C., Eshwara, V. K., Bhat, P., Acharya, S., Kamath, A., Bhat, S., et al., (2016). Risk factors for preterm birth and low birth weight among pregnant Indian women: A Hospital-based Prospective Study. *Journal of Preventive Medicine and Public Health*, 49: 165-175.

[43] Lohana, M. H., Suragimath, G., Patange, R. P., Varma, S., Zope, S. A. (2017). A prospective cohort study to assess and correlate the maternal periodontal status with their pregnancy outcome. *Journal of Obstetrics and Gynecology of India*, 67: 27-32.

[44] Abati, S., Villa, A., Cetin, I., Dessole, S., Luglie, P. F., Strohmenger, L., Ottolenghi, L., & Campus, G. G. (2013). Lack of association between maternal periodontal status and adverse pregnancy outcomes: a multicentric epidemiologic study. *The Journal Of Maternal-fetal & Neonatal Medicine : The Official Journal Of The European Association Of Perinatal Medicine, The Federation Of Asia And Oceania Perinatal Societies, The International Society Of Perinatal Obstetricians*, 26: 369–372.

[45] Guimarães, A. N., Silva-Mato, A., Miranda Cota, L. O., Siqueira, F. M. & Costa, F. O. (2010). Maternal periodontal disease and preterm or extreme preterm birth: an ordinal logistic regression analysis. *Journal of Periodontology*, 81: 350-358.

[46] Giannella, L., Giulini, S., Cerami, L. B., La Marca, A., Forabosco, A. & Volpe, A. (2011). Periodontal disease and nitric oxide levels in low risk women with preterm labor. *European Journal of Obstetrics Gynecology and Reproductive Biology*, 158: 47-51.

[47] Piscoya, M. D. B. V, Ximenes, R. A. A., Silva, G. M., Jamelli, S. R. & Coutinho, S. B. (2012). Maternal periodontitis as a risk factor for prematurity. *Pediatrics International*, 54: 68-75.

[48] Macedo, J. F., Ribeiro, R. A., Machado, F. C., Assis, N. M. S. P., Alves, R. T., Oliveira, A. S. & Ribeiro, L. C. (2014). Periodontal disease and oral health-related behavior as factors associated with preterm birth: a case-control study in South-Eastern Brazil. *Journal of Periodontal Research,* 49: 458-464.

[49] Martinez de Tejada, B., Gayet-Ageron, A., Combescure, C., Irion, O. & Baehni, P. (2012). Association between early preterm birth and periodontitis according to USA and European consensus definitions. The Journal Of Maternal-fetal & Neonatal Medicine: The Official Journal Of The European Association Of Perinatal Medicine, The Federation Of Asia And Oceania Perinatal Societies, *The International Society Of Perinatal Obstetricians 25,* 3: 2160-2166.

[50] Nabet, C., Lelong, N., Colombier, M. L., Sixou, M., Musset, A. M., Goffinet, F. & Kaminski, M. (2010). Maternal periodontitis and the causes of preterm birth: The case-control Epipap study. *Journal of Clinical Periodontology,* 37: 37-45.

[51] Iwanaga, R., Sugita, N., Hirano, E., Sasahara, J., Kikuchi, A., Tanaka, K. & Yoshie, H. (2011). FcγRIIB polymorphisms, periodontitis and preterm birth in Japanese pregnant women. *Journal of Periodontal Research,* 46: 292-302.

[52] Bulut, G., Olukman, O. & Calkavur, S. (2014). Is there a relationship between maternal periodontitis and preterm birth? A prospective hospital-based case-control study. *Acta Odontologica Scandinavica,* 72: 866-873.

[53] Jain, S., Sharma, S., Chawla, S., Vaid, B. N., Kalra, N., Suneja, A., Guleria, K. & Kaur, L. (2016). Periodontal disease as a risk factor for preterm delivery in Indian women. *J. Evolution Med. Dent. Sci,* 5: 6565-6569.

[54] Chaparro, A., Sanz, A., Quintero, A., Inostroza, C., Ramirez, V., Carrion, F., Figueroa, F., Serra, R. & Illanes, S. E. (2013). Increased inflammatory biomarkers in early pregnancy is associated with the development of pre-eclampsia in patients with periodontitis: a case control study. *Journal of Periodontal Research,* 48: 302-307.

[55] Hirano, E., Sugita, N., Kikuchi, A., Shimada, Y., Sasahara, J., Iwanaga, R., Tanaka, K. & Yoshie, H. (2012) The association of Aggregatibacter actinomycetemcomitans with pre-eclampsia in a subset of Japanese pregnant women. *Journal of Clinical Periodontology,* 39: 229-238.

[56] Moura da Silva, G., Coutinho, S. B., Piscoya, M. D. B. V, Ximenes, R. A. A. & Jamelli, S. R. (2012). Periodontitis as a risk factor for pre-eclampsia. *Journal of Periodontology,* 83: 1388-1396.

[57] Ide, M. & Papapanou, P. N. (2013) Epidemiology of association between maternal periodontal disease and adverse pregnancy outcomes – systematic review. *Journal of Periodontology,* 84: S181-S194.

[58] Vettore, MV, Lamarca, GA., Leão AT., Thomaz FB., Sheiham A., Leal MC,. (2006). Periodontal infection and adverse pregnancy outcomes: a systematic review of epidemiological studies. *Cad. Saúde Pública, Rio de Janeiro,* 22: 2041-2053.

[59] Corbella S. Tascheri S, Fabrro M, Francetti L, Weinstein R, Ferrazzi E. (2018). Adverse pregnancy outcomes and periodontitis: A systematic review and meta-analysis exploring association. *Quintessence international,* 47: 193 – 204.

[60] Vivares-Builes, A. M., Rangel-Rincón, L. J., Botero, J. E., Agudelo-Suárez, A. A. (2018). Gaps in knowledge about the association between maternal periodontitis and adverse obstetric outcomes: an umbrella review. *J Evid Based Dent Pract,* 18: 1–27.

[61] Teshome, A., Yitayeh, A. (2016). Relationship between periodontal disease and preterm low birth weight: systematic review. *Pan African medical journal,* 24: 215 – 224.

[62] Correder, E. D., Beltran, D. O., Pineda, A. L., Queseda, J. A., Guillen, V. F., Munuera, C. C. (2019). Maternal periodontitis and preterm birth: Systematic review and meta-analysis. *Community dentistry and oral epidemiology,* 47; 243 – 51.

[63] Sayafer, I. F., Tahir, H., Oktawati, S. (2019). The correlations between periodontal disease in the woman with pregnancy and low

birth weight infant: a systematic review. *Makssan Dental Journal,* 8: 12-21.

[64] Daalderop, L. A., B. V. Wieland, K. Tomsin, L. Reyes, B. W. Kramer, S. F. Vanterpool, and J. V. Been. (2018). Periodontal Disease and Pregnancy Outcomes: Overview of Systematic Reviews. *JDR clinical and translational research,* 3: 10 – 27.

[65] Corbella, S., M. Del Fabbro., S. Taschieri., L. Francetti. (2012). Periodontal disease and adverse pregnancy outcomes: a systematic review. *Italian Oral Surgery,* 11: 132-146.

[66] Kim, J. A., Lo, A. J., Pullin, D. A., Johnson, D. S., Karimbux, N. Y. (2012). Scaling and Root Planing Treatment for Periodontitis to Reduce Preterm Birth and Low Birth Weight: A Systematic Review and Meta-Analysis of Randomized Controlled Trials. *J Periodontol,* 83: 1508 – 19.

[67] Oliveria, L. P., Fontanari, A., Chaves, A., Coasta, M. R., Cirelli, J. A. (2010). Effect of periodontal treatment on the incidence of preterm delivery: a systematic review. *Minerva Stomatol,* 62: 1-2.

[68] Schwenicke, F., Karimbux, N., Allareddy, V., Gluud, C. (2015). Periodontal Treatment for Preventing Adverse Pregnancy Outcomes: A Meta- and Trial Sequential Analysis. *PLoS One,* 10: e0129060.

[69] Bi, W. G., Emami, E., Luo, Z. C., Santamaria, C., Wei, S. Q. (2019). Effect of periodontal treatment in pregnancy on perinatal outcomes: a systematic review and meta-analysis. *The Journal of Maternal-Fetal & Neonatal Medicine,* 5: 1-10.

[70] Fogacci. M., Fampa, M. S. C., Vettore, M., Vianna, M., Leão, T., Thereza, A., (2011). The Effect of Periodontal Therapy on Preterm Low Birth Weight: A Meta-Analysis. *Obstet and Gynaecol,* 117: 153 – 165.

[71] Uppal, A., Uppal, S., Andres, P., Dutta, M., Shrivatsa, S., Dandolu, V., Mupparapu, M. (2010). The Effectiveness of Periodontal Disease Treatment during Pregnancy in Reducing the Risk of Experiencing Preterm Birth and Low Birth Weight: A meta-analysis. *The Journal of the American Dental Association,* 11: 1423-1434.

[72] Rosa M., Ines M., Simões PD., Medeiros., Rosi L., Isabe, M., Jeovany, M. M., (2012). Periodontal disease treatment and risk of preterm birth: a systematic review and meta-analysis. *Cadernos de Saúde Pública*, 28: 1823-1833.

BIOGRAPHICAL SKETCH

Jananni Muthu

Affiliation: Associate professor, Department of Periodontology, Indira Gandhi Institute of Dental Sciences, Sri Balaji Vidyapeeth, Deemed to be university, Pondicherry, India.

Education: MDS, PGDHPE.

Research and Professional Experience:

- Teaching experience:
- 7 years of postgraduate teaching
- 3 years' experience as dental educator
- 10 completed research projects, 3 ongoing research projects, 1 funded research project

Professional Appointments:

- Associate professor at Department of Periodontology, Indira Gandhi Institute of Dental Sciences, Sri Balaji Vidyapeeth, Deemed to be university, Pondicherry, India
- Managing director, Smile studio, Dental Clinic, Pondicherry.
- Adjunct faculty, Centre for Health Professions education.

Honors:

Awards	
1	Merit award by Indian Society of Pediatric and Preventive dentistry for securing first mark in Pediatric dentistry in Final year BDS examinations 2009
2	Third place in poster presentation at Givadent, Perio CDE at Annamalai University - 2012
3	Third place in poster presentation at Colgate lecture series, Meenakshi Ammal Dental College & Hospital, Chennai
4	Best faculty team presentation award at ISP national conference at Kochi, 2013
5	Cash award for publication in high impact journal at SBV, Pondicherry - 2017
6	Third place in paper presentation at SBV research week, Pondicherry - 2017
7	Best faculty paper presentation award at TIMS conference, Annamalai University, Chidambaram - 2018
8	Special prize for faculty paper presentation at SBV research week, Pondicherry - 2019
9	Cash award for publication in high impact journal at SBV, Pondicherry - 2017

Recognitions			
S. no	Type of recognition	Details	Date
1	Peer reviewer	Association of periodontal inflammation with glycemic control in patients with type 2 diabetes" (ID - FMD-2015-0068)in the journal" Frontiers of medicine"	September 2015
2	Resource person	Training of trainers program organized by IGIDS for internal faculty	Sep 2015
3	Guest lecture	Lecture in Perio Nexux – Colgate lecture series	29.9.2015
4	Resource person	Training of trainers program organized by DEU for faculty from Karpaga Vinayaka Institute of Dental Sciences, Chennai	January 2016
5	Peer reviewer	"Assessment of oral health attitudes and behavior among students of Kuwait University Health Sciences Center" in the journal "Journal of International society of public health & community dentistry"	June 2016
6	Resource person	Training of trainers program organized by DEU in Priyadarshini Dental College & Hospital, Chennai	June 2016

7	Peer reviewer	Editorial board member – EC Dental Science	2016
8	Peer reviewer	Editor – Case reports - Journal of Scientific dentistry	2016
9	Peer reviewer	Peer reviewer – Journal of International Society of Public health & community dentistry	2016
10	Peer reviewer	Peer reviewer – Journal of endocrinology & metabolism	2016
11	Resource person	Resource person for PG pedagogy program held at IGIDS and presented on the topic "Teaching & learning media"	21.9.2016
12	Resource person	Resource person for TOTS FDP program held on at PDCH, Chennai and presented on the topic "Teaching & learning media"	13.6.2016
13	Editorial board member	EC Dental Science	2017
14	Section editor	Journal of Scientific dentistry	2017
15	Peer reviewer	Peer reviewed articles in Journal of Current Vascular Pharmacology	2017
16	Peer reviewer	Reviewed article in Journal of Oral Health and Dental Sciences	2017
17	Key note speaker	"Scope of periodontology" at Chettinad Dental college	7.03.2017
18	Resource person	TOTS, SRM dental college, Chennai	1.3.2017
19	Peer reviewer	Reviewed article in Journal of Indian Society of Public and Community Dentistry	2017
20	Peer reviewer	Reviewed article in Journal of Chronic Diseases and Management	2017
21	Editorial board member	EC Dental Science	2018
22	Section editor	Journal of Scientific dentistry	2018
23	Peer reviewer	Peer reviewed article in Integrated clinical and medical case reports	2018
24	Peer reviewer	Peer reviewed article in Journal of Epidemiology & Global Health	2018
25	Peer reviewer	Peer reviewed articles in Journal of Basic clinical and applied health sciences	2018
26	Peer reviewer	Peer reviewed articles in Journal of Oral Health and Dental Sciences	2018

27	Resource person	Do,s and Don'ts of powerpoint at BICS class at IGIDS	12.10.2018
28	Certificate of appreciation	IQAC certificate of appreciation	2018
29	Peer reviewer	Peer reviewed article in International journal of Oral & Dental Health	2018
30	Promotion	Promoted as Reader	30.10.2018
31	Certificate of appreciation	Certificate of appreciation for Hon LG, Dr. Kiran Bedi	2018
32	Editorial board member	– EC Dental Science	2019
33	Peer reviewer	Peer reviewer for Frontiers of Medicine	2019
34	Peer reviewer	Peer reviewer for Journal of Dentists	2019
35	Peer reviewer	Peer reviewer for Applied Biologic Research	2019
36	Peer reviewer	Peer reviewer for Journal of Orofacial Research	2019
37	Guest lecture	Special lecture on the topic Biofilm formation as a part of Indian Society of Periodontology's Listerine series of Lectures	02.08.2019
38	Resource person for TOTS 1	Empowering teaching expertise	Feb 2019
39	Peer reviewer	Peer reviewed article in Frontiers of Medicine	2019
40	Chairperson	Chaired a scientific session in "Perio Sakthi" National CDE, APDCH, Melmaruvathur.	(13.9.2019)
41	Resource person	Resource person – Listerine series of lectures (ISP) at IGIDS	02.08.2019
42	Peer reviewer	Peer reviewed article in the Journal of Dentists	2019
43	Peer reviewer	Peer reviewed article in Applied Biologic Research	2019
44	Peer reviewer	Peer reviewed article in Journal of Orofacial Research	2019
45	Invited observer	Observer for IHRC Yoga workshop	21.7.2019
46	Certificate of appreciation	Certificate of appreciation for 4 copyrights during SBV research week	28.1.2019
47	Chair person	Chaired a scientific session at Perioparadigms – International conference on changing trends and innovations in periodontology	17.11.2019

Publications from the Last 3 Years:

1. Muthu, J., Muthanandam, S., Sethuraman, K. R, Narayan, K. A, Ananthakrishnan, N., Adkoli, B. V. 2019. Assessment of Self Perception of Competencies among a Group of Dental interns in Pondicherry, India. *J Educ Health Promot.* 8: 255. Pubmed.
2. Muthu, J., Sivaramakrishnan, M., Mahendra, J., Syed, K., Maher, F., Khair, M. 2019. Periodontitis presage pre-diabetes – A comparative study of glycemic control in non-diabetic population with and without periodontal disease. *Biomedicine,* 39(4): 595- 598. Pubmed, Scopus.
3. Sivaranjani. K. S., Balu, P., Kumar, R. S., Muthu, J., Devi, S. S., Priyadharshini, V. 2019. Correlation of periodontal status with perceived stress scale score and cortisol levels among transgenders in Puducherry and Cuddalore. *SRM J Res Dent Sci,* 10: 61-4. Google scholar.
4. Kumar, B. Na., Balu, P., Muthu, J., Kumar, R. S., Karthikeyan, I., Devi, S. S. 2019. Correlation of stress and periodontal disease severity among coal mine workers in Tamilnadu: A clinicobiochemical study. *Indian J Multidisip Dent,* 9: 36-39. Google scholar.
5. Muthu, J., Sivaramakrishnan, M., Kuduruthullah, S. S. K., Fattah, M. A., Kaseh, A. E. L., Khair, M. B., Fathy, E. K. 2019. Orthodontic Button Assisted Coronally Advanced Flap for Treatment of Multiple Teeth Recession: A Case Report with Literature Review. *World J Dent,* 10: 35 - 39. Scopus.
6. Gayathri, E., Indrakumar, S. P., Saravanakumar, R., Muthu, J., Pratebha, B. 2019. Periodontal screening and recording versus traditional Clinical periodontal examination in the assessment of periodontal status. *Int J Sci Res,* 8(4): 1-5. Google Scholar.
7. Muthu, J., Sivaramakrishnan, M. 2018. Periodontitis and respiratory diseases: What does the current evidence point to? *Current Oral Health Reports,* 5: 63 – 9. Pubmed.

8. Muthu, J., Sivaramakrishnan, M., Kuduruthullah, S., Fateh, M. A. 2018. A novel technique for multiple teeth recession coverage – Modified semilunar coronally advanced flap. *Int J Sci Res*, 10: 68-70. Pubmed.
9. Ughabharathy, R., Balu, P., Muthu, J., Saravanakumar, R., Vineela, K., Karthikeyan, I. 2018. Clinical evaluation of increase in the width of attached gingiva using modified apically repositioned flap: A 9-month follow-up study. *Contemp Clin Dent*, 9: 200-4. Pubmed.
10. Ahila, E., Saravana Kumar, R., Reddy, V. K., Pratebha, B., Muthu, J., Priyadharshini, V. 2018. Augmentation of interdental papilla with platelet-rich fibrin. *Contemp Clin Dent*, 9: 213-7. Pubmed.
11. Arvina, R., Pratebha, B., Saravana Kumar, R., Muthu, J. 2018. Assessment of true end points in periodontal flap surgery patients –A DIDL questionnaire study. *Journal of basic, clinical and applied health sciences,* 2: 25-30. Google scholar.
12. Aravind Raaj, V., Muthu J., Pratebha, B., Saravanakumar, R., Vineela, K., Sakthi Devi, S. 2018. Light Microscopic Analysis of Toothbrush Bristle End Morphology - An In Vitro Study. *Acta Scientific Dental Sciences,* 2: 84-88. Google scholar.
13. Muthu, J., Sivaramakrishnan, M., Umapathy, G., Kannan, A. L. 2017. Fibrotic encapsulation of orthodontic appliance in palate. *Journal of Indian Society of Periodontology,* 21(5):427-428. Pubmed.
14. Elangovan, G. P., Mutu, J., Periyasamy, I. K., Balu, P., Kumar, R. S. 2017. Self-reported prenatal oral health-care practices of preterm low birth weight-delivered women belonging to different socioeconomic status: A postnatal survey. *J Indian Soc Periodontol*, 21:489-93. Pubmed.
15. Kuduruthula, S., Muthu, J., Sivaramakrishnan, M. 2017. Short term, low dose Amlodipine induced severe gingival enlargement – A case report. *International Journal of current research*, 5: 51179 – 82. Google scholar.
16. Muthu, J., Sivaramakrishnan, M., Jaideep, M. 2016. Mouth the mirror of lungs – Where does the connection lie? *Front. Med*, 10(4): 405–409. Pubmed, Scopus.

INDEX

A

acid, vii, ix, 58, 62, 83
active transport, 63, 64
age, viii, 2, 3, 6, 8, 10, 11, 13, 14, 31, 39, 47, 48, 50, 53, 54, 55, 63, 73, 76, 77, 81
air pollutants, 49
alcohol consumption, viii, 2, 23, 25, 41, 42, 50, 90
alcohol use, 41
alkaline phosphatase, 61
amniotic fluid, 60, 85
antibody, 83
antioxidant, 71
anxiety, 5, 19, 37
appointments, 50
artery, 68, 70, 71
autonomic nervous system, 20

B

bacteria, 80, 82, 83, 84, 85, 91
bacterial infection, 84
bacterial pathogens, x, 79
behaviors, 14, 47, 50, 81
beneficial effect, 72, 89
biochemistry, 77
biomarkers, 35, 68, 75, 95
birth rate, viii, 2, 3, 10, 11, 13, 14, 20, 23, 47, 48, 49, 50
birth weight, x, 33, 35, 41, 42, 48, 53, 54, 55, 80, 81, 84, 86, 87, 88, 89, 90, 93, 94, 96, 97, 103
births, viii, ix, 2, 3, 5, 7, 12, 13, 14, 19, 26, 28, 33, 37, 42, 48, 51, 52, 53, 54, 55, 57, 59, 60
birthweight, 38, 55
black women, 14, 48
blood, 15, 16, 35, 65, 69, 70, 76, 77
body mass index, 36
bone, ix, 58, 59, 61, 62, 63, 64, 65, 66, 67, 68, 69, 70, 72, 73, 74, 75, 76, 77, 93
bone form, 61, 63, 64, 65, 68, 69, 71, 72, 75, 77
bone marrow, 62
bone mass, 74
bone mineral content, ix, 58, 59, 66
bone resorption, x, 58, 61, 62, 63, 64, 65, 68, 69, 72, 74

bone turnover, 57, 58, 61, 63, 64, 65, 67, 69, 71, 72, 74, 76
breast milk, 65, 66, 69
breastfeeding, 7, 65, 67

C

calcitonin, 64, 65, 67
calcium, 63, 64, 65, 66, 67, 77
carbon monoxide, 22
cardiovascular diseases, x, 80
Caucasian population, 15
cell line, 49
cell signaling, 15
central nervous system, 71
cervical intraepithelial neoplasia, 8, 30
cervix, 8, 20, 29, 30
child mortality, 26
childhood, 63, 65, 74
children, viii, 2, 3
cigarette smoking, 39, 40
circulation, 63, 82, 85
community, 8, 27, 52, 89, 99, 100
complications, viii, ix, 2, 3, 7, 10, 11, 17, 26, 46, 50, 60, 85, 92, 93
conception, 4, 6, 11, 12, 20, 25, 28, 32, 40, 49
cone biopsy, 29
conference, 99, 101
consumption, 18, 23, 37, 41, 42, 68, 75
contaminated water, 16
control group, 12, 69
controlled studies, 32
controversial, 23, 24
controversies, ix, 58, 59
conversion rate, ix, 58
correlation, 13, 15, 16, 17, 18, 20, 22, 23, 47, 49, 87
cytokines, x, 20, 58, 61, 62, 68, 83, 85, 86, 92
cytoplasm, 86

D

deaths, viii, 2, 3, 20, 46, 59
defense mechanisms, 83
demographic characteristics, viii, 2, 53
depressive symptoms, 19
depth, vii, viii, 2, 8, 30
destruction, 82, 83
detection, ix, 8, 58, 59, 84, 91
developed countries, 14, 59
diabetes, x, 80, 81, 102
dilatation and curettage, 9, 30
diseases, x, 61, 73, 80, 81, 82, 91, 102
docosahexaenoic acid, vii, ix, 58, 75
docosahexaenoic acid (DHA), v, vii, ix, 57, 58, 67, 68, 70, 72, 73, 75
drug abuse, 42
drugs, 14, 18, 24

E

economic status, 10, 11, 13, 15, 16, 17, 24
educated women, 50
education, 15, 47, 48, 98
educational attainment, 14, 34
eicosapentaenoic acid, vii, ix, 58, 75
electromagnetic, 55
electromagnetic fields, 55
employment status, 58
endocrinology, 73, 74, 76, 100
enlargement, 82, 103
environment, 21, 25, 47, 60
environmental tobacco, 22
epidemiologic, vii, viii, 2, 35, 46, 88, 94
epidemiologic studies, 35, 88
epidemiology, 2, 26, 28, 42, 46, 96
epidemiology of preterm birth, 2, 26, 27, 46, 77
ethnicity, viii, 2, 14, 82
etiology, viii, x, 46, 47, 79
exposure, 16, 35, 37, 40, 42, 49, 54, 55

F

fatty acids, vii, ix, 18, 37, 58, 62, 70, 73, 75
fertilization, 53
fetal development, 39, 47, 67
fetal distress, ix, 46, 52
fetal growth, 22, 41, 52, 91
fetal risk factors, 46, 47, 51
fetus, 46, 63, 64, 66, 74, 75
fibroblast growth factor, 70
fish oil, ix, 18, 58, 68
formation, 61, 62, 63, 64, 65, 69, 70, 101

G

gender differences, 56
gene expression, 72
genes, 15, 50, 86, 93
genetic background, 5
genetic components, 47
genetic predisposition, 93
gestation, vii, ix, 1, 2, 3, 4, 8, 9, 12, 13, 38, 41, 51, 57, 59, 63, 64, 67, 71, 72, 73, 90
gestational age, vii, ix, 1, 2, 4, 6, 8, 13, 34, 35, 39, 40, 41, 42, 43, 54, 57, 59, 60, 66, 70, 76, 90
gestational diabetes, 10
gingival, 81, 82, 89, 103
growth, 43, 61, 62, 64, 65, 67, 70
growth factor, 61, 62, 64, 70

H

health, ix, x, 4, 14, 16, 19, 21, 25, 35, 38, 39, 47, 58, 68, 75, 77, 80, 89, 92, 93, 100, 103
health care, 25
health effects, 35
health promotion, 58
heart disease, 80

heart rate, 35, 60
high school degree, 49
higher education, 14, 50, 58
high-risk women, 8
history, viii, 2, 4, 8, 9, 20, 27
homeostasis, 70, 73
homocysteine, 18, 37
hormones, 36, 61, 62, 69, 74
human, ix, 38, 51, 58, 75, 92
human development, 75
human leukocyte antigen, 51
hyperparathyroidism, 64, 67
hypertension, 10, 61, 81

I

iatrogenic, 10, 11, 15, 18, 21, 51
identification, 25
imbalances, 61
immersion, 75
immune response, 83, 86
immune system, viii, 46, 47, 71
incidence, viii, 8, 14, 19, 39, 46, 47, 52, 60, 66, 88, 89, 97
income, viii, 2, 10, 14, 16
infants, ix, 11, 12, 14, 15, 51, 52, 55, 57, 59, 66, 76, 77, 87, 88, 92, 94
infection, 12, 20, 60, 82, 83, 84, 85, 86, 89, 91, 92, 96
inflammation, x, 15, 16, 35, 76, 80, 82, 85, 92, 99
inflammatory bowel disease, 86
inflammatory disease, x, 79, 80
inflammatory mediators, 83, 84, 85
intrauterine growth retardation, 31, 41

L

lactation, 63, 64, 65, 68, 69, 70, 72, 73
learning, 4, 100
learning difficulties, 4

leiomyoma, 28
leiomyomata, 28
leptin, 68, 69, 73, 76
low birthweight, 41, 42, 54
low risk, 90, 94

M

marital status, viii, 2, 18, 19, 37
maternal risk factors, viii, 2, 4, 46
maternal smoking, 60
matrix, 62, 63, 66, 83
mechanical ventilation, 60
medical, viii, 2, 9, 10, 53, 60, 89, 96, 100
medicine, viii, x, 2, 59, 73, 76, 80, 99
membranes, viii, x, 1, 4, 7, 15, 20, 34, 41, 71, 80, 84, 86, 93
menstruation, 40
mesenchymal stem cells, 68
meta-analysis, 4, 6, 7, 16, 22, 26, 27, 29, 30, 34, 40, 93, 96, 97, 98
metabolism, ix, 58, 63, 66, 68, 69, 70, 71, 72, 73, 74, 75, 76, 77, 100
mineralization, 61, 65, 66, 67, 70, 72
morbidity, viii, 2, 3, 25, 46, 51, 52, 58, 81
mortality, 3, 25, 51, 52, 58, 81, 89
multivariate analysis, 19

N

neonate, v, ix, 2, 3, 57, 58, 59, 66, 67, 68, 69, 71, 72, 74
nutrition, 65, 72, 75, 76, 77
nutritional deficiencies, ix, 58, 59, 61
nutritional status, 81

O

omega-3, vii, ix, 58, 68, 69, 70, 71
oral cavity, x, 79, 82

oral health, 95, 99, 103
osteoclastogenesis, 62
osteopenia, vii, ix, 57, 59, 66, 74
osteoporosis, ix, 58, 65, 74, 75, 76, 80
oxidative stress, 16, 35

P

paternal risk factors, vii, ix, 46, 47, 54
paternal support, 47, 49
pathophysiological, viii, 46, 47
pathophysiology, 47, 69
perinatal, 7, 15, 29, 31, 40, 42, 54, 59, 89, 97
periodontal, x, 79, 80, 82, 83, 84, 85, 86, 87, 88, 89, 90, 91, 92, 93, 94, 96, 97, 99, 102, 103
periodontal disease, x, 79, 80, 82, 84, 86, 87, 88, 89, 90, 91, 93, 94, 96, 102
periodontal flap surgery, 103
periodontitis, vii, x, 80, 84, 86, 87, 88, 91, 92, 93, 94, 95, 96
phosphorus, 63, 64, 66, 67, 72, 75
placenta, 21, 63, 83, 84, 86
placental abruption, 22, 34
polyunsaturated fat, ix, 58, 75, 76
polyunsaturated fatty acids, ix, 58, 75, 76
population, 6, 14, 15, 16, 17, 28, 33, 38, 55, 62, 90, 102
positron emission tomography, 38
pregnancy, vii, x, 2, 3, 5, 6, 7, 8, 9, 10, 11, 12, 13, 14, 17, 18, 19, 21, 22, 23, 24, 26, 27, 28, 29, 30, 32, 36, 37, 38, 39, 40, 41, 42, 43, 47, 50, 53, 55, 58, 60, 63, 64, 65, 67, 70, 72, 73, 76, 77, 80, 81, 82, 83, 84, 85, 86, 87, 88, 89, 90, 91, 92, 93, 94, 95, 96, 97
premature contraction, 6
premature infant, 66
prematurity, ix, 3, 32, 39, 55, 57, 58, 59, 60, 66, 76, 94

preterm delivery, viii, 15, 19, 32, 33, 37, 38, 39, 40, 41, 42, 46, 54, 55, 95, 97
preterm infants, ix, 57, 59, 60, 72, 74
preterm neonates, 48, 58, 59
prostaglandin, 21, 62, 72, 77, 92
psychological distress, 36
psychological problems, 81
psychological stress, 19

R

reproductive age, 6, 24
requirements, 61, 65, 70, 72
response, x, 23, 41, 62, 65, 66, 79, 81, 84, 85, 86
risk, vii, viii, ix, x, 2, 4, 5, 6, 7, 8, 9, 10, 11, 12, 13, 14, 15, 17, 18, 19, 21, 22, 23, 24, 25, 26, 27, 28, 29, 30, 31, 32, 33, 34, 36, 37, 38, 39, 40, 41, 42, 46, 47, 48, 49, 50, 51, 52, 53, 54, 55, 58, 59, 65, 72, 80, 81, 82, 84, 85, 88, 89, 92, 93, 94, 95, 96, 98
risk factors, vii, viii, 2, 4, 14, 15, 18, 24, 25, 26, 46, 47, 52, 81, 82, 85, 88

S

sex, ix, 46, 47, 51, 52, 55, 56, 64, 67
sex steroid, 64, 67
sexual activity, 19
skeleton, 61, 62, 63, 65, 67, 70
smoke exposure, 22
smoking, viii, 2, 15, 18, 21, 22, 24, 25, 39, 40, 47, 50, 81, 82
social environment, 3
social problems, 24
social support, 19
socioeconomic status, 17, 48, 58, 103
stillbirth, 33, 55, 81, 84
stress, 19, 20, 21, 25, 27, 35, 36, 38, 39, 47, 50, 53, 82, 85, 90, 102
stressful events, 20

stressful life events, 20, 38
supplementation, 68, 69, 70, 71, 72, 73, 74
survival rate, ix, 2, 3, 57, 59
syndrome, viii, 3, 7, 25, 28, 46, 47
synthesis, 38, 62, 64, 66, 70

T

therapeutic interventions, 61
therapy, 88, 89
tissue, 18, 61, 83, 84, 93
TNF-α, x, 58, 68
tobacco smoke, 22, 40
treatment, ix, x, 8, 11, 16, 30, 58, 60, 80, 88, 89, 97, 98
trial, 9, 10, 16, 19, 41, 48, 49, 50, 51, 74
tumor necrosis factor, 91
turnover, 58, 61, 64, 65, 69, 71, 72, 74, 76
type 1 diabetes, 74
type 2 diabetes, 99

U

umbilical cord, 68, 69, 70, 71
uterine fibroids, 6, 28
uterus, 5, 6, 52, 63, 67, 86

V

vein, 68, 69, 70, 71
vitamin D, 61, 63, 64, 67
vulnerability, 76

W

workers, 35, 102
working conditions, 39

ω

ω-3 PUFA, ix, 58